YOUR GUIDE TO GOOD NUTRITION

YOUR GUIDE TO GOOD NUTRITION

FREDRICK J. STARE, M.D.
VIRGINIA ARONSON, M.S., R.D.
STEPHEN BARRETT, M.D.

PROMETHEUS BOOKS • BUFFALO, NEW YORK

Published 1991 by Prometheus Books

95 94 93 92 91   5 4 3 2 1

Library of Congress Cataloging-in-Publication Data

Stare, Fredrick J. (Frederick John), 1910–
    Your guide to good nutrition / Frederick J. Stare, Virginia Aronson, Stephen Barrett.
        p.   cm.
    Includes index.
    ISBN 0-87975-692-6
    1. Nutrition. I. Aronson, Virginia. II. Barrett, Stephen, 1933–   . III. Title.
RA784.S74   1991
613.2—dc20   91-27297
                                                                    CIP

Printed in the United States of America on acid-free paper.

Contents

1 A Taste of Nutrition Basics 1

2 Balancing Your Diet 16

3 How to Evaluate Nutrition Information 26

4 Vitamin and Mineral Supplements 47

5 "Health Foods" and Other Magic Potions 60

6 "Junk Foods" and "Fast Foods" 87

7 The Truth about Additives 95

8 Practical Weight Control 110

9 Healthy Vegetarian Eating 132

10 The Truth about Sugar 141

11 Fluid Facts 150

12 Tips for Teenagers 162

13 Diet, Heart Disease, and Cancer 171

Appendix A. Recommended Dietary Allowances 185

Appendix B. Glossary 187

Appendix C. Recommended Reading 198

Index 202

Introduction

Every day you eat food, as you have been doing all of your life. You know that diet is important to health and well-being. Do you feel that you know enough about basic nutrition? Do you understand your own dietary needs? The actual components of your daily diet? Which foods are "good" for you? And whether there are any "bad" foods? Do you wonder whether our food supply is unsafe? Whether the latest weight-loss diet would work for you? And whether your diet will contribute to your health and longevity?

These issues hang heavily on the minds of today's consumers. Everywhere you turn, you face more dietary advice: newspapers, billboards, bookstores, supermarkets, magazines, restaurants, radio and television ads, and talk shows are all making food claims, yet few promote the same dietary concepts. Upon whom can you rely to answer your nutrition questions and steer you down the road toward a healthful diet?

Your Guide to Good Nutrition was written in response to the pressing need for a reliable and easy-to-understand book on nutrition for laypersons. Follow its advice to add to your health, protect your pocketbook, and increase your eating pleasure.

Fredrick J. Stare, M.D., Ph.D.
Virginia Aronson, R.D., M.S.
Stephen Barrett, M.D.

About the Authors

• Fredrick J. Stare, M.D., Ph.D., is Professor Emeritus of Nutrition and founder of Harvard University's Department of Nutrition. He is also cofounder and a board member of the American Council on Science and Health. He was a member of the Food and Nutrition Board of the National Research Council for many years, and has served as consultant to numerous voluntary and governmental agencies, food companies and trade associations. One of the world's most prominent nutritionists, he has received awards from seven major professional societies.

Dr. Stare is author or coauthor of sixteen books, more than four hundred research and review articles in peer-reviewed scientific journals, and many other articles in lay publications. He was, for twenty-five years, editor of the prestigious journal *Nutrition Reviews*. He wrote a nationally syndicated newspaper column for nearly forty years and has also moderated a syndicated radio program. His books include *Balanced Nutrition: Beyond the Cholesterol Scare; Eating for Good Health; Living Nutrition; Eat OK—Feel OK; The Harvard Square Diet; Panic in the Pantry;* and *The 100% Natural, Purely Organic, Cholesterol-Free, Megavitamin, Low-Carbohydrate Nutrition Hoax*. His most recent book is an autobiography titled *Adventures in Nutrition*.

• Virginia Aronson, R.D., M.S., is a nutritionist and professional writer. She serves on the editorial board of the American Running and Fitness Association and has contributed many articles to professional and lay publications. Her eleven books include five with Dr. Stare (*Your Basic Guide to Nutrition, Food for Today's Teens, Rx: Executive Nutrition, Food for Fitness and Fifty,* and *Dear Dr. Stare: What Should I Eat?*); three textbooks (*Guidebook for Nutrition Counselors, Thirty Days to Better Nutrition,* and *The Dietetic Technician: Effective Nutrition Counseling*); and the *I-Don't-Eat-But-I-Can't-Lose Weight Loss Program,* written with triathlete/physician Steve Jonas. In 1988 she coauthored White House Chef Henry Haller's *The White House Family Cookbook.* Her latest project is a book describing the link between creativity and mental health.

• Stephen Barrett, M.D., who practices psychiatry in Allentown, Pennsylvania, is a nationally renowned author, editor, and consumer advocate. An expert in medical communications, he edits *Nutrition Forum Newsletter* and is medical editor of Prometheus Books. He also contributes regularly to *Priorities Magazine, Healthline Newsletter,* and *Consumer Reports Health Letter.* He is a board member of the National Council Against Health Fraud and chairs its Task Force on Victim Redress. His twenty-seven books include *The Health Robbers; Vitamins and "Health" Foods: The Great American Hustle; Consumer Health—A Guide to Intelligent Decisions;* and *Health Schemes, Scams, and Frauds.* In 1984 he won the FDA Commissioner's Special Citation Award for Public Service in fighting nutrition quackery. In 1986 he was awarded honorary membership in the American Dietetic Association. In 1987 he began teaching health education at The Pennsylvania State University.

Acknowledgements

The authors are grateful to the following individuals for their many helpful suggestions during the preparation of the manuscript:

Project manager   Robert Basil, Senior Editor, Prometheus Books
Proofreader   Jacob Nevyas, Ph.D., Allentown, Pennsylvania
Technical editor   Manfred Kroger, Ph.D., Professor of Food
                       Science, The Pennsylvania State University

1

A Taste of Nutrition Basics

Think for a moment about driving a car. Good drivers understand the rules of the road and use good judgment in driving. When your car needs repair, some knowledge of the car's mechanics can make you a wiser *consumer* of these services. But it is not necessary to understand a car's inner workings to be a good *driver*.

Similarly, it is not necessary to know a great deal about the science of nutrition in order to eat properly. To achieve optimal nutrition, one must follow the basic rules of good *eating*. Some knowledge of nutritional biochemistry and human physiology can help you recognize which rules to follow to be a wise *consumer*, but good eating actually requires little knowledge of what happens to foods within your body.

What are the basic
"rules" of good nutrition?

The basic principles of good nutrition are *variety, balance,* and *moderation.* Wise food selection can be made by following the guide-lines in Chapter 2 of this book. These guidelines are quite simple to follow. Weight control can be achieved by exercising regularly and controlling portion sizes (particularly of foods that are high in fat), as discussed in Chapter 8. This might not be so easy to do, but there are no safe shortcuts to achieving a reasonable body weight.

1

Let's return to our car analogy. Suppose you are driving from New York to California. There are countless routes you can take. You may consider which routes are shortest, most scenic, or safest. You may want to visit certain people or places along the way. You may want to take some toll roads and not others. The length and quality of the trip may also be affected by the weather, the mechanical condition of your car, the speed at which you drive, road conditions, any passengers you take, and many other factors. With a good road map and travel plan, you will probably enjoy your trip and reach California.

Suppose, however, that your map is inaccurate or misleading—and that road signs along the way have been tampered with to beckon you in the wrong direction. If you obtain a better map and are perceptive enough to ignore the phony signs, you will reach your destination efficiently. If not, you may become anxious and confused, and your trip may be longer, more costly—and even dangerous. This situation is comparable to that faced by consumers who seek to travel the road to good nutrition. The scientific facts form a clear path for the nutritionally knowledgeable, but the constant flow of misinformation to the public creates roadblocks for others attempting to find the way.

How can I tell whose advice to follow?

Your best bet is to be guided by qualified health professionals who advocate methods based on the collective wisdom of the scientific community. This wisdom is based upon the "scientific method," a set of logical rules to determine which theories and methods are valid and which are not. This approach—which combines accurate observations with appropriate statistical analysis—has enabled medical science to conquer many diseases that were rampant centuries ago. Chapter 3 tells how to identify professionals who base their practices on scientific rules.

What nutrients have scientists determined that we need?

The chemical elements essential to life include hydrogen, oxygen, carbon, and nitrogen—which together make up about 98 percent of most forms of life and food—and about twenty minerals. *Water* is formed from hydrogen and oxygen. *Carbohydrates* and *fats* are formed from hydrogen, oxygen, and carbon. *Proteins* are formed from hydrogen, oxygen, carbon, and nitrogen. *Vitamins* are composed of carbon, hydrogen, and oxygen; most also contain nitrogen, and a few contain sulfur.

The essential chemical elements combine to form about fifty nutrients essential for human life. The six basic categories of these nutrients are listed in Table 1:1. With a few exceptions, these nutrients are not manufactured in the body and must be obtained through dietary intake. Proteins, carbohydrates, and fats are the only nutrients that can provide the body with energy (calories), while vitamins, minerals, and water do not provide any calories but are necessary for the body to process foods that do contain them. Ethyl alcohol, in alcoholic beverages, also provides calories; but alcohol is more appropriately regarded as a drug rather than a food.

Table 1:1. Basic Categories of Essential Nutrients

Macronutrients (large amounts needed; supply body energy)

Protein components (amino acids): isoleucine, leucine, lysine, methionine, phenylalanine, threonine, tryptophan, valine; histidine (only for infants)

Carbohydrate: glucose

Fat: linoleic acid

Micronutrients (small amounts needed; regulate body functions)

Vitamins: vitamin A, vitamin D, vitamin E, vitamin K, thiamin, riboflavin, niacin, pantothenic acid, folacin, vitamin B_6, vitamin B_{12}, biotin, vitamin C

Minerals: arsenic, boron, calcium, chloride, chromium, cobalt, copper, fluoride, iodide, iron, magnesium, manganese, molybdenum, nickel, phosphorus, potassium, selenium, silicon, sodium, sulfur, zinc

Water

How can I tell how much of these nutrients I need?

A committee of the Food and Nutrition Board of the National Research Council confers periodically to review the scientific studies bearing on this question. Their recommendations—called Recommended Dietary Allowances (RDAs)—are updated and published periodically—usually about every five years. The RDAs are the levels of intake of essential nutrients "adequate to meet the known nutrient needs of practically all healthy persons." Appendix A lists the current (1989) values for Americans at all age levels.

There are RDAs for protein, eleven vitamins, and seven minerals. It is important to understand that RDAs are guidelines primarily intended for use in evaluating the nutrient intake of population groups. RDAs are not *minimum* daily requirements, but include rather large margins of safety. They are set high enough to allow for individual variations. Intakes equivalent to half of the RDAs are usually adequate.

Are the RDAs considered "optimal amounts" for good health?

Little or no data exist for determining what levels of individual nutrients might be "optimal." The RDAs—by definition—encompass what is known about the need for individual nutrients. They are intended to be high enough—even allowing for variability within the total population—so that no health benefit should be expected from increasing intakes above RDA levels. Relationships between dietary patterns and disease, which are a separate matter, are addressed by the U.S. Dietary Guidelines, which we cover in Chapter 2. Some people claim that large doses of vitamins, minerals, and amino acids can play a role in the prevention of many diseases. However, the vast majority of nutrition scientists do not support this viewpoint.

Many essential nutrients are not listed in the RDA tables. Why not?

If your daily diet contains adequate amounts of the key nutrients listed in the RDA tables, you are also likely to be receiving adequate amounts of those not listed in the tables.

Food labels refer to "U.S. RDAs." What are they?

Food labels state the percentage of U.S. RDA per serving of food for each nutrient present in significant amounts. The U.S. RDAs (U.S.

Recommended Daily Allowances) are based on the 1968 RDA table, in most cases using the highest level for each life-cycle category. In 1990 the FDA announced a proposal to replace the U.S. RDAs with a new system of "Reference Daily Intakes (RDIs)" based on the 1989 RDAs. These values will still be more than what most people need.

Other requirements for food labels are undergoing intensive review by the FDA and are likely to change within the next year or two. Regardless, if you are on a special diet or need help with careful dietary analysis, you probably should enlist the aid of a registered dietitian or other qualified nutritionist who provides nutrition counseling (see Chapter 3).

Is it necessary to memorize Table 1:1 and the RDAs in order to make wise food choices?

No! Nor is it necessary to analyze every mouthful you eat to be sure you meet the RDA for each given nutrient. Chapter 2 describes the Basic Four Food Group system, which classifies foods according to their major nutrient characteristics. Following this system will automatically provide the nutrients needed by healthy persons. Ailing individuals with special nutrient needs (such as people who are unable to absorb certain nutrients through their intestinal tract) should have professional guidance. Anyone who advises healthy persons to take doses of vitamins and minerals higher than the RDAs "to be sure they get enough" is bypassing the collective wisdom of the scientific nutrition community.

What happens to foods within the body?

The digestive tract—also called the gastrointestinal tract or alimentary canal—provides the pathway through which foods move through the body. During this process, foods are broken down into their component nutrients to be available for absorption.

Digestion actually begins in the mouth, as the enzymes in saliva begin to break down carbohydrate (starch). As food is chewed, it becomes lubricated, warmer, and easier to swallow and digest. The teeth and mouth work together to convert each bite of food into a bolus that can readily move into the esophagus ("the food pipe"). In the meantime, taste buds located in the mouth help you to enjoy each mouthful—or to find the food distasteful, as is sometimes the case. After the bolus is swallowed, it enters the esophagus where it

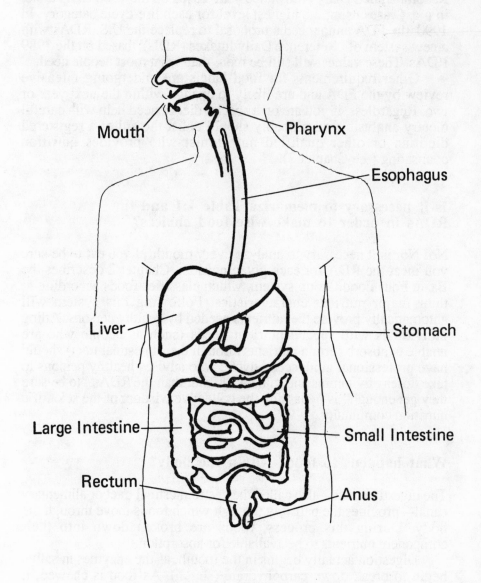

THE DIGESTIVE SYSTEM

continues to be warmed and lubricated as it moves toward the stomach.

The acidic environment of the stomach and the action of gastric enzymes convert the bolus into chyme, a liquefied mass that is squirted from the stomach into the small intestine. Carbohydrates tend to leave the stomach rapidly and enter the small intestine; proteins leave the stomach less rapidly; and fats linger there the longest.

The small intestine is the principal site of digestion and absorption. There, enzymes and secretions from the pancreas, liver, gallbladder, and the small intestine itself combine to break down nutrients so that they can be absorbed. The pancreas is a veritable enzyme factory, supplying enzymes to digest proteins, fats, and carbohydrates. Intestinal cells also supply some enzymes. The liver produces the bile required for the emulsification of fat, and the gallbladder stores the bile until it is needed. The absorption of nutrients in the small intestine is facilitated by tiny projections called villi, which provide more surface area for absorption. The nutrients pass through the intestinal membranes into the circulatory system, which transports them to body tissues. Nutrients are then absorbed into the cells, where they are used for growth, repair, and the release or storage of energy. The overall process—called *metabolism*—is highly complex.

Undigested chyme proceeds from the small intestine into the large intestine (colon), where it becomes concentrated, as liquid is absorbed in preparation for excretion. Bacteria cause fermentation, which facilitates further breakdown, but absorption of nutrients from the large intestine is minimal.

The key point to remember about digestion is that foods must be broken down into their component nutrients before they can be absorbed. Since so-called "health foods" do not contain any nutrients that cannot also be found in a varied and balanced diet of "ordinary" foods, it is easy to understand why scientists regard the concept of "health foods" as meaningless.

Now let's examine a few more biochemical facts that can help you steer clear of any misinformation you may encounter.

Proteins

Proteins differ from carbohydrates and fats because, in addition to the carbon, hydrogen, and oxygen that comprise the last two, proteins also contain nitrogen. The nitrogen is incorporated into the structure of the subunits of protein called amino acids. Eight of some twenty-two amino acids used by the adult body are essential and must be obtained from food, while the rest can either be obtained from food or made within the body. Both plant and animal foods contribute protein to the diet, but, except for gelatin, only animal protein contains all eight of the essential amino acids. During digestion, food proteins are broken down and absorbed as their component amino acids—which are then used to build proteins within the body. Proteins can also be used for energy if sufficient amounts of fat or carbohydrate are not available. Most Americans consume considerably more protein than they need.

Carbohydrates

Carbohydrates can be divided into two groups: those digestible by humans (glucose, other sugars, and starches), and the indigestible ones (cellulose, pectin, and gums), referred to collectively as "fiber." Almost exclusively the product of plants, carbohydrates are excellent sources of energy for the body. If carbohydrate is not supplied in the diet, the body must make glucose from fat or protein, which is a less efficient process.

Glucose has been called "the universal sugar" because it is the basic form of food energy for life—for both humans and plants. Foods must be broken down by the body into glucose before the energy within them is accessible. Cellulose can be used for energy by cattle, other ruminating (cud-chewing) animals, and termites, but the human body cannot break down indigestible carbohydrates, which are largely excreted. Although the indigestible carbohydrates are not used by the body for energy, fiber is important to good health for other reasons.

Glucose is a single sugar unit (monosaccharide), as are fructose and galactose. The double sugars (disaccharides) are: maltose (malt sugar), composed of two glucose molecules; lactose (milk sugar), composed of glucose plus galactose; and sucrose (table sugar), composed of glucose plus fructose. Single and double sugars are termed "simple" sugars. They can be used rapidly for energy or stored for later use.

How is energy stored?

Starch is the common mode of energy storage used by plants, while humans and other animals store most of their energy as fat and a small amount as glycogen, a form of starch. Starches, which are also called "complex carbohydrates," are composed of long chains of glucose molecules. To provide energy, the chains must be broken down to glucose. Proteins can also be broken down to glucose. Glycogen is stored mainly in the liver and the muscles.

Fat is a more concentrated energy storage form than glycogen. Unfortunately for some of us, the body can store rather extensive supplies of energy in its fat cells. This fuel, which may never be needed, must then be carried around by its overfat proprietor.

Why are these carbohydrate facts significant?

Many misinformed individuals believe that sucrose is dangerous— even "poisonous"—and that complex carbohydrates are safer and more desirable. It is true that foods containing complex carbohydrates (and fiber) are an important part of a balanced diet. But it is ridiculous to claim that one type of digestible carbohydrate is dangerously inferior to the others when all become glucose in the body anyway. All edible carbohydrates are safe when eaten in moderate amounts.

Fats

Lipid is a chemical term for fatty substances, including triglycerides (fats and oils), phospholipids (such as lecithin), and sterols (such as cholesterol). In common usage, fats are lipids that appear solid at room temperature, while oils are lipids that are liquid at room temperature. The term "triglyceride" is frequently used when discussing food fats in general, and triglycerides are the most common form of fat found in the body. Triglyceride molecules are composed of glycerol (an alcohol) plus three chainlike fatty acids.

Linoleic acid, a fatty acid, is the only fat component recognized as an essential nutrient for humans. Lipids in the diet actually contain many other fatty acids, but since these can be synthesized from other substances, they are not considered essential. Fatty acids differ in the length of their chains and their degree of saturation with hydrogen. Those filled to capacity with hydrogen are called "saturated" fatty acids, while those with room for two more hydrogen atoms are called "monounsaturated" fatty acids. Those with room for four or more hydrogen atoms are called "polyunsaturated" fatty acids (PUFAs). Linoleic acid is a PUFA and is found mainly in certain plant oils.

Triglycerides can contain combinations of fatty acids of all types: short chains, medium chains, long chains, saturated, mono-unsaturated, and/or polyunsaturated. The dominant type of fatty acid determines the characteristics of the triglyceride. Oils tend to be rich in polyunsaturates whose many points of unsaturation are vulnerable to the spoiling capabilities of oxygen. Thus, oils will eventually become rancid with exposure to air. Two vegetable oils, palm oil and coconut oil, are mostly saturated. Most saturated fats are of animal origin, or are vegetable oils that have been made more saturated (e.g., oleomargarine) by a commercial process called hydrogenation. Since saturated fats are less vulnerable to rapid spoilage, they are used in processed foods to prolong shelf life.

Chapter 13 provides information on the relationship between dietary fats, cholesterol, and heart disease.

Vitamins

Chemical substances that contain carbon are termed "organic." Vitamins are organic substances required in very small amounts to promote one or more specific biochemical reactions within the living cell. There are thirteen vitamins for humans. Four are fat-soluble (A, D, E, and K), and nine are water-soluble (C and the eight "B-complex" vitamins: thiamin, niacin, riboflavin, pantothenic acid, folacin, B_6, B_{12}, and biotin). Vitamins are catalysts—substances that initiate or speed up chemical reactions but remain unchanged while performing their tasks repeatedly. This explains why only tiny amounts are needed by the body.

Vitamins perform a wide range of functions in the body. They do not provide energy directly to the body, but most are part of the enzyme systems required for the release of energy from carbo-hydrates, fats, proteins, and alcohol. Vitamins are also required for the synthesis of many essential body compounds, such as enzymes and hormones. Normal growth and maintenance of body tissues depend on an adequate supply of vitamins.

Why does it matter whether vitamins are fat-soluble or water-soluble?

Fat-soluble vitamins are not excreted efficiently by the body. They are generally stored in body fat until they are used, and thus can accumulate to toxic levels. Excess amounts of water-soluble vitamins do not build up in this manner but are excreted in the urine. Excesses of both types can have adverse effects (see Chapter 4), but the fat-soluble vitamins tend to be more dangerous.

About twenty years ago, the FDA proposed that nutrient supplements at doses 1½ times the U.S. RDA or more be classified and regulated as drugs. But a massive political campaign by vitamin and "health food" promoters prevented this regulation from being implemented.

Are there any significant differences between "natural" vitamins and synthetic ones?

No. A few synthetic vitamins are slightly different in structure from their natural counterparts, but these differences have no practical significance. The body cannot tell the difference between "natural" and synthetic varieties. In the marketplace, however, the "natural" label usually commands a higher price. So it is being applied not only to vitamins and foods, but to a wide range of products—including cosmetics, beer, and even cigarettes.

In 1974, the Federal Trade Commission (FTC) began wrestling with the idea of regulating the use of the words "natural," "organic," and "health" in food advertising. The agency's first inclination was to ban them, but protests from supporters of these terms changed this plan. For a time, it appeared that the FTC might create a legal definition of the word "natural" despite warnings from scientists that any definition would be meaningless and misleading. The rulemaking procedure was abandoned in 1983 as part of the Reagan Administration's philosophy of making government "less intrusive."

The words "natural," "organic," and "health" are emotionally powerful slogans. But don't let yourself be hoodwinked into paying higher prices for them! They are three road signs to ignore along the road to good nutrition.

Minerals

Minerals are inorganic (not carbon-containing) compounds needed in relatively small amounts by the body. They do not supply the body with fuel, but many act as catalysts for the release of energy from carbohydrates, fats, proteins, and alcohol. Minerals also help regulate many bodily functions and foster the growth and maintenance of body tissues.

About twenty minerals are now considered essential for humans. The major minerals (macrominerals) are those present in the body in amounts exceeding five grams: calcium, phosphorus, chloride, potassium, sulfur, sodium, and magnesium. The rest are known as trace minerals, or microminerals.

Which minerals are most significant for consumers?

For some segments of the population, certain minerals are in short supply in the diet, while others are consumed in more than adequate amounts. Those that may not be included in sufficient quantities in the diet are iron, fluoride, calcium, and sometimes potassium. Americans tend to take in excessive amounts of sodium.

Iron

Most Americans are familiar with iron, largely because of advertisements about "tired" or "iron-poor" blood. Iron is a key ingredient in hemoglobin, the red pigment responsible for assisting in the transport of oxygen in the blood. In iron-deficiency anemia, the red blood cells carry less oxygen to body tissues, resulting in pallor and general fatigue. This problem is common in the United States—particularly in low-income groups—in infants, children, women of childbearing age, and the elderly.

Iron deficiency can occur with blood losses such as the constant low-grade bleeding caused by ulcers, parasites, or some types of cancer. The condition can also be caused by a diet low in iron. Since iron is not well absorbed from food, it is difficult for some people to follow a diet that prevents the development of iron deficiency. Animal sources of iron (liver and other red meats, poultry, and fish) are better absorbed than plant sources (dried peas and beans, spinach and other dark green leafy vegetables, whole grain and enriched breads and cereals, dried fruits and their juices). Vitamin C enhances iron absorption, and cooking in iron cookware can increase iron content of foods. On the other hand, high-fiber diets may reduce iron absorption, largely due to the presence of components that can bind minerals and render them inabsorbable (less bioavailable).

Growing children, young women, pregnant women, vegetarians, and other susceptible individuals should try to consume a diet that includes plenty of iron-rich foods, but a physician may prescribe a supplement if iron deficiency is diagnosed.

Fluoride

When the natural concentration of fluoride is too low in a community's water supply, individuals raised in the area will suffer from considerably more tooth decay than people from areas with adequate amounts of fluoride in their water. Fluoride may also play a role in the prevention or delay of osteoporosis, a condition in which the bones become porous and brittle. Most foods are not good sources of this mineral, but fish with bones that are eaten (such as sardines) and tea can contribute some fluoride to the diet.

The process of adding fluoride to a community water supply is called fluoridation. Close to 130 million Americans now live in communities served by naturally or artificially fluoridated water. Unfortunately, despite oceans of evidence showing that fluoridation is safe, effective, and economical, controversy has prevented implementation in many communities. Children raised in nonfluoridated communities should be given supplementary fluoride, as discussed in Chapter 4.

In areas where the fluoride content of water is naturally excessive, mottling of the teeth may occur in individuals who consume such water prior to six or seven years of age. In such areas, defluoridation to the proper level is desirable.

Calcium

Calcium—along with fluoride and vitamin D—is essential for the proper formation and maintenance of bones and teeth. About 99 percent of this major mineral is found in these two body parts, while less than 1 percent is involved in the equally important functions of nerve transmission, muscle contraction (including the beating of the heart), blood clotting, and maintenance of connective tissue (collagen).

Deficiency of calcium in children causes the bone deformity disease called rickets and a similar disorder in adults known as osteomalacia. (These conditions are usually caused by poor absorption of calcium because of lack of vitamin D rather than insufficient calcium in the diet.) Osteoporosis is a common disease in the aged—especially in women—in which the total amount of bone decreases. Although hormonal imbalances may be more important than diet in the development of osteoporosis, the significance of maintaining adequate intakes of dietary calcium, fluoride, and vitamin D should not be overlooked.

Milk is our most common source of calcium, but cheese, yogurt, and other foods made with milk also provide significant amounts of this essential mineral. When eaten with the bones, sardines and canned salmon are rich in calcium. Dark green leafy vegetables such as spinach and broccoli contain significant amounts of calcium, but in a less absorbable form. If dairy products are eliminated, it is difficult to construct a diet containing adequate amounts of absorbable calcium.

Potassium

This mineral plays an important role in the maintenance of a steady heartbeat and is essential for proper fluid balance. Potassium is also required by the nervous system and for the metabolism of other nutrients. Potassium deficiency sometimes occurs in people who use certain diuretics (see Chapter 4) or follow a restrictive diet (see Chapter 8). Excessively high levels of potassium in the blood can cause serious trouble, so potassium supplements should never be used without medical supervision.

Sodium

There rarely occurs a shortage of sodium in the diet. This mineral is readily absorbed and is plentiful in foods. Essential for fluid balance, nerve transmission, and muscle contraction, the sodium content of body tissues is usually regulated carefully. During a period of heavy sweating, the body can become dehydrated, flushing out considerable amounts of sodium as well as water. Overly rigid sodium restriction can also deplete the body's supply of this mineral. Fortunately, a few shakes of the salt shaker can easily replenish sodium levels.

Some individuals with high blood pressure are "sensitive" to sodium. In these persons, a sharp reduction in sodium intake will lower blood pressure. This is discussed further in Chapter 13.

Water

Water is involved in all chemical reactions in the body, including the release of energy from carbohydrates, fats, proteins, and alcohol. Water also acts as a medium for the transport of nutrients, and as a lubricant. The evaporation of water from the lungs and skin is a vital aspect of body temperature control. Water is available not only in beverages, but also in many foods, particularly fruits and vegetables, where it may constitute 80 to 90 percent of these commodities. Water's overall importance is highlighted by the fact that an individual will become ill and die much faster from a lack of water than from a deficiency of any other nutrient.

Fueling the human machine

Like a modern car, the human body is a highly complicated machine. Fortunately, to make our bodies operate smoothly, most of us need only provide the proper fuel—as calories plus essential nutrients in the form of a well balanced diet. To guide yourself down the road to good nutrition, however, you must carefully evaluate the signs you encounter along the way. Some will reflect the science of nutrition and the facts on sensible eating, while others will tempt you with pseudonutritional nonsense. The following chapter can help you to fuel up properly for the journey to good health.

2

Balancing Your Diet

No single food contains the fifty or so nutrients that the body requires in amounts adequate for proper growth and health. All the nutrients we need, however, can be provided by foods. A well balanced diet contains the proper array of nutrients. Since foods vary in the kinds and amounts of nutrients they provide, it is important to consume a variety of foods each day.

Is it true that people in this country were better nourished during our grandparents' time and that our diets have gradually become worse?

Absolutely not! According to recent surveys and diet studies of individuals, groups, and families, as well as information compiled by the U.S. Department of Agriculture from "food disappearance" data, Americans are now more adequately nourished as a population than they were at the turn of the century. In fact, we are better nourished than any other people in the world at any time in history. These days, people who are ill-fed are either ignorant, negligent, or too poor to buy the food they need. Since all the essential nutrients are readily available, people who are not well nourished cannot honestly blame their dietary inadequacies on today's food supply.

With over 20,000 different food items now available in the typical supermarket, how can the average shopper make proper food choices?

Actually, a well balanced (and tasty) diet is quite simple to achieve. Nutritionists have incorporated both the bodily needs of individuals and the nutritive values of foods into what is called the Basic Four Food Groups system of classification. Each group contains a variety of foods with similar nutrient composition. You can ensure an adequate intake of essential nutrients by including in your daily diet the recommended number of servings from each of the four groups. For best results it is advisable to choose a variety of foods within each group and to moderate the intake of fats.

Is the "Basic Four" concept outdated?

Definitely not! The Basic Four guidelines still provide the easiest way to plan for adequate nutrition on a daily basis by encouraging people to eat a variety of foods that will provide a balanced diet. Although not structured to enumerate all of the foods encountered daily, the Basic Four Food Groups provide a simple, practical framework for menu planning. Total caloric intake can be controlled by adjusting portion sizes, especially for high-calorie foods like meats and whole-milk dairy products.

The four basic groups are: Fruit & Vegetable Group, Grain & Cereal Group, Milk & Cheese Group, and Meat & Alternates Group. Sweeteners and fats are included in the Basic Four only as ingredients of other foods (e.g., breakfast cereals that contain sugar can be Grain & Cereal Group selections).

Most people include plenty of sugar and fat in their daily diet. Like sugar, alcoholic beverages don't provide vitamins or minerals but are potent sources of calories. To decrease your caloric intake, first cut back on foods high in fat and on alcoholic beverages.

How does the Basic Four system work?

Tables 2:1 and 2:2 illustrate the food groups, recommended servings, food sources, nutrient contributions, and major nutrient functions. You may want to place copies of these charts in a handy spot in your kitchen so that you can easily refer to them when planning menus or preparing shopping lists. Soon the information they provide will

become second nature to you, and eating based on the Basic Four
Food Groups will become a daily habit.

Table 2:1. Basic Four Food Groups
Serving sizes, particularly of the Milk and Meat groups, should be
adjusted appropriately to reach and maintain desirable weight.

Basic Food Group	Recommended No. Daily Servings	Serving Size	Food Sources
Fruit & Vegetable	4	1/2 cup cooked 1/2 cup juice 1 cup raw	Fruit or juice, including citrus frequently. Dark green leafy or bright yellow vegetables 3-4 times weekly
Grain & Cereal	4	1 slice 1/2–3/4 cup 1/2 cup	Breads: whole-grain and enriched, muffins, rolls, tortilla Cereals: cooked, dry, whole-grain, rice, grits, barley flours, millet, buckwheat Pasta: macaroni, noodles, spaghetti Starchy vegetables: corn, lima beans, peas, potato, pumpkin, winter squash
Milk & Cheese	2 (adult) 3 (child) 4 (teen)	1 cup 1 1/2 oz. 1–1 3/4 cup	Milk, yogurt Cheese (calcium content greater in harder varieties) Milk-containing foods
Meat & Alternates	2	2–3 oz. 1 2 tbsp. 1/2 cup 1 cup	Meat, poultry, fish Eggs Peanut butter, nuts* Cottage cheese Dried beans and peas*

*For an acceptable meat alternative, combine with animal protein
(Meat & Alternates Group or Milk & Cheese Group foods) or with
Grain & Cereal Group selection.

Table 2:2. Major Nutrient Groups

Nutrient	Major Functions in Body	Best Food Sources
Protein 4 calories per gram	Forms cell structure; supports growth, maintenance, and repair of tissue; needed for enzymes and hormones	Meat & Alternates Group Milk & Cheese Group
Carbohydrate 4 calories per gram	Serves as primary energy source; can provide fiber for proper digestive function	Grain & Cereal Group Fruit & Vegetable Group
Fat 9 calories per gram	Serves as concentrated energy source; supplies essential fatty acid; carries fat-soluble vitamins	Milk & Cheese Group: whole milk products Meat & Alternates Group: meats, nuts, peanut butter Other sources: butter, margarine, oils, salad dressing, fried foods, and many processed foods
Vitamins & Minerals	Perform various functions to help regulate body processes; necessary in order to obtain energy from foods	Fruit & Vegetable Group: vitamins A, C Grain & Cereal Group: B vitamins Milk & Cheese Group: calcium, phosphorus, riboflavin Meat & Alternates Group: B vitamins, iron
Water	Transports nutrients; helps regulate body temperature; aids in digestion	Water Other fluids Fruit & Vegetable Group Milk & Cheese Group: milk

What about the Dietary Guidelines?

In 1980 and 1985, the U.S. Department of Agriculture and the Department of Health and Human Services published a booklet describing seven general guidelines for decreasing the odds of developing certain chronic diseases. After expert review, the guidelines were revised slightly and reissued in 1990, as follows:

1. Eat a variety of foods.
2. Maintain healthy weight.
3. Choose a diet low in fat, saturated fat, and cholesterol.
4. Choose a diet with plenty of vegetables, fruits, and grain products.
5. Use sugars in moderation.
6. Use salt and sodium in moderation.
7. If you drink alcoholic beverages, do so in moderation.

These guidelines amplify the principles of variety, balance, and moderation inherent in the Basic Four Food Group system. Some experts believe that the guidelines should also call attention to consuming adequate amounts of fluoride (to prevent tooth decay) and calcium (to help prevent osteoporosis). Though not mentioned in the guidelines themselves, these points are discussed in the guidelines booklet. A free copy can be obtained by requesting *Dietary Guidelines for Americans* (HG232) from Consumer Information Center, Dept. 514-X, Pueblo, CO 81009.

I understand that the U.S. Surgeon General and National Research Council have issued nutrition guidelines. Are they similar?

Yes. The 750-page *Surgeon General's Report on Nutrition and Health* (1988) and the 996-page National Research Council report, *Diet and Health* (1989), offer thorough scientific analyses of the relationships between diet and the occurrence of chronic diseases. Their recommendations are similar to the Dietary Guidelines but include much more detail.

Are these various guidelines applicable to children?

Consistent with the fact that children below the age of two are not "little adults," the Gerber Products Company has published guidelines modeled after the 1985 *Dietary Guidelines for Americans* and based on published statements by the American Academy of Pediatrics' Committee on Nutrition. The guidelines are:

• *Build to a variety of foods.* Unlike adults, infants do not require a variety of foods to secure nutrition during the first six months or so of life. Human milk alone provides the vitamins, minerals, carbohydrates, fats, and proteins needed for normal growth and development during early infancy. Except for fluoride, vitamin D (in the absence of adequate exposure to sunlight), and occasionally vitamin K, supplements to human milk are not required during this period. Infant formula is recommended as the best alternative to human milk if breastfeeding is not used or is stopped early. Most babies are ready to start supplemental foods around four to six months of age. Single-grain cereal is often the first food added after breast milk or formula. Other single-ingredient foods can be added gradually until the baby is eating a variety of foods.

• *Listen to your baby's appetite to avoid overfeeding or underfeeding.* Although healthy infants can vary considerably from one another in their caloric intake, appetite is likely to be the most efficient way to determine what an infant needs. Babies should be fed when they are hungry but should not be forced to finish the last few ounces of formula in a bottle or spoonfuls of food in a dish.

• *Don't restrict fat and cholesterol too much.* Although low-fat and low-cholesterol diets are widely recommended for adults, they are not appropriate for infants under the age of two. Infants require fat in their diet to satisfy needs for normal growth and development.

• *Don't overdo high-fiber foods.* Infants and small toddlers eating a well-rounded diet probably get enough fiber for their needs. A diet high in fiber may be too low in calories and may interfere with absorption of iron, calcium, magnesium, and zinc.

• *Sugar is okay, but in moderation.* Sugar, which exists in several forms, is a source of calories and makes some foods taste better. Breast milk, the ideal food for infants, contains lactose, which is similar to table sugar. Other foods in a balanced diet may contain moderate amounts of sugar, but excessive amounts of such foods can crowd out more nutritious foods.

• *Sodium is okay, but in moderation.* Although the amount of sodium in the diet of a small percentage of adults is related to high blood pressure, the amount of sodium in an infant's diet has not been shown to cause high blood pressure in later life. Even though healthy infants can tolerate a range of sodium intakes without ill effects, moderation in sodium intake is urged.

• *Babies need more iron, pound for pound, than adults.* Infants are born with a stored supply of iron that lasts for the first four to six months of life. Iron is more likely than any other nutrient to be lacking in the infant diet. For this reason, special efforts should be made to provide infants with iron during the first two years. The best sources are iron-fortified formula and iron-fortified infant cereal.

Two versions of the Gerber guidelines have been published, a 20-page booklet for consumers and a 36-page booklet for health professionals. Either can be obtained free of charge by calling Gerber's consumer information center at 1-800-4-GERBER.

Why are carbohydrates the main source of energy in the world's diet?

Partly because of economics. Foods rich in carbohydrates tend to be less expensive than those high in protein or fat. Also, carbohydrate is the body's ready form of energy. Although often considered fattening and "the dieter's number-one enemy," carbohydrate is lower in calories than is typically believed. It provides only 4 calories per gram (115 calories per ounce), as does protein. Fat, however, provides 9 calories per gram (255 calories per ounce), while alcohol provides 7 calories per gram. Carbohydrate-rich foods deserve popularity because many can provide us with essential nutrients, fiber, and ready energy without adding to our waistline.

Do individuals active in sports require more protein than non-athletic individuals?

Americans tend to overemphasize the importance of protein and to eat two to three times the amount required for good health. Many athletes hold misconceptions about diet and tissue-building and believe that a very large protein intake will lead to bigger and better muscles. This is simply not true. The protein requirement for athletes is readily met—and often exceeded—simply by eating a normal diet.

Is it true that only food fat turns into body fat?

No. Carbohydrates, proteins, fats, and alcohol are the body's only sources of energy. Energy is measured in calories. An excess of calories from any source (including alcohol) will be stored in the body as fat. Fat, however, is the most concentrated source of calories. Thus, small amounts of fat can contribute significant amounts of calories. It's not the baked potato (carbohydrate) that is high in calories, but the sour cream or butter (fat) spread on top!

Some fats are visible (e.g., butter, margarine, and oils), but some are hidden in foods (e.g., meats, cheese, milk, eggs, nuts, fried foods, and many processed foods). The fat content of meat products can be surprisingly high, as illustrated in Table 2:3.

An excessive intake of calories from any type of food will lead to weight gain. Loss of weight can be facilitated, however, if fatty foods are limited and replaced in part by fruits, vegetables, and other low-fat foodstuffs.

Table 2:3. Fat Content of Some Meats

Food and Amount	Total No. of calories	No. Calories from fat	% Calories from fat
Porterhouse steak, 10.6 oz.	1400	1136	80
T-bone steak, 10.4 oz.	1395	1140	82
Corned beef, 4 oz.	422	311	74
Ham, 5.5 oz.	576	424	74
Pork chops, 2.7 oz.	305	222	73
Spareribs, 6.3 oz.	792	560	71
Bologna, 1 oz.	86	70	81
Sausage, brown-and- serve, 1 link	83	68	82
Frankfurter, 1 (2 oz.)	176	141	80
Salami, 1 oz.	128	97	76
Bacon,* 2 slices	86	70	82

*Considered a fat serving rather than a Meat & Alternates Group item.

How much can we rely on protein as an energy source?

Carbohydrate, protein, and fat are the three food sources of calories, but the body relies mainly on carbohydrate and fat. Protein can furnish calories when the intake of carbohydrate and fat is low, but protein is also necessary for making body proteins such as muscle tissue, enzymes, and hormones. Thus, when proteins are used to provide energy, their building functions are impeded. Alcohol is another source of calories, although most people don't think of it as a food.

I have felt tired and run-down lately. Do I need to take some kind of a multivitamin and mineral supplement?

Probably not. Surveys have found that most American adults believe that extra vitamins promote "pep" and energy, and generally lead to better health. The truth, however, is that carbohydrates, proteins, and fats are the nutrient sources of energy. Vitamins and minerals are noncaloric. They do not supply energy directly but enable the body to use the energy provided by food. Eating a well balanced diet that includes moderate amounts of a variety of foods chosen from the Basic Four Food Groups (including variety within each group) should provide all the vitamins the body needs. If you are unusually tired, see a physician. It is likely that your problem is not nutritional in nature but is due to physical or emotional factors. It might even be caused by something as easily remedied as insufficient sleep.

How much water do I need every day?

Water is a nutrient we tend to forget about. Yet water is our most important nutrient, second only to air as essential for the maintenance of life itself. The human body requires about one quart of water for every 1,000 calories consumed, or about six to eight glasses per day. This requirement varies with the weather and degree of physical activity. Water does not come only from the tap, but is present in differing amounts in most foods. Most fruits and vegetables, for example, are 80 to 90 percent water.

How has the American diet changed during the past fifty years or so?

Some major changes in the nutritional status of Americans have occurred during the past half-century, and there have been a number of modifications in eating patterns as well. Although isolated cases of the classic nutritional deficiency diseases (such as rickets, scurvy, beriberi, and pellagra) still occur, the clear-cut nutritional diseases that once plagued this country have practically disappeared. Instead, Americans have developed other nutritional problems, mostly as a result of eating and drinking more than they need.

Data from national nutritional surveys indicate that caloric intake has remained relatively constant, rising only slightly over the years, but the amount of physical activity necessary to use up these calories has declined. The proportion of calories derived from protein has changed little since 1910, but the protein sources have changed. While grain and other vegetable sources once provided half of our protein, today about 70 percent comes from animal products. Overall consumption of carbohydrates has declined during this century, and the sources have changed; the consumption of flour and grain products has declined, while total sweetener consumption has increased. Vitamin and mineral intakes have not diminished during this century. In fact, the levels of calcium, vitamin C, and vitamin A in the food supply are higher today than they were fifty years ago. The enrichment of flour, bread, and cereal products has added other nutrients to the modern food supply.

The total fat intake of American consumers has remained about the same, but because carbohydrate intake has decreased, the relative proportion of fat has increased slightly. Fortunately, the types of fat consumed have changed. During the last two decades, we have consumed less lard, butter, and whole milk, substituting more margarine, vegetable oils, and low-fat milk. Yet our generous consumption of meat still contributes to excessive intake of saturated fats.

Our main dietary problem now is not a lack of good food, but the tendency to eat too much of it! Modern technology has made available a varied, nutrient-rich, tasty, and exciting menu. It is up to us as informed consumers to choose foods wisely. This can be done by eating a variety of items from among and within the Basic Four Food Groups—with portions of high-calorie foods and beverages adjusted to maintain a reasonable body weight.

3

How to Evaluate Nutrition Information

Nutrition has always been a popular topic for faddists and quacks. Throughout history, misguided and misinformed individuals have warned the public about dietary dangers and claimed that eating special foods could cure illness and extend the human lifespan. Since nutrition science has developed relatively recently, it is not hard to understand the persistent popularity of diet mythology.

Nor is it difficult to understand why people today are seduced by nutrition misinformation. Although careful consumers can avoid falling prey to nutrition quackery, recognizing a diet hoax can be difficult. Advocates of quack methods, many of whom are sincere in their beliefs, may represent themselves as acting in the public interest when they are actually exploiting public hopes and fears, or seeking personal economic gain.

Today's "health food" industry is a multibillion dollar business that promotes a multitude of products that supposedly can prevent and cure the gamut of human ailments. Health food stores are fountainheads of misinformation. Multilevel companies such as Shaklee and Amway have convinced thousands of Americans to peddle nutrition products to their friends. Bookstore shelves overflow with paperbacks describing all sorts of nutritional schemes such as "crash" weight-loss plans, "anti-aging" diets, and "miracle" cures. Nonfiction bestseller lists usually contain at least one diet or nutrition book that would be more appropriately listed as fiction.

Radio and television talk shows abound with self-appointed "experts" spreading erroneous nutrition advice to unsuspecting audiences. And even some major pharmaceutical companies use scare tactics to promote unnecessary vitamins.

Consumers beware! Few Americans are undernourished. Not many illnesses are primarily diet-related, and only a few are curable through diet alone. Our food supply is basically safe and can easily provide the nutrients we need. Popular reducing diets are rarely based on scientific principles, and few prove beneficial in the long run.

Are you looking for magic from nutrition? Or are you seeking the facts? This chapter can help you separate nutrition myths from facts, and it also tells how to recognize a nutrition quack.

How do you define quackery?

A simple definition would be "that which claims too much in the field of health." William T. Jarvis, Ph.D., Professor of Health Education at Loma Linda University, stresses that quackery involves *promotion for profit.* ("Quacks quack," he says.) He also notes that "quackery lies in the promise, not the product." Thus a product (such as a vitamin) that has legitimate uses becomes a vehicle for quackery when promoted with false or misleading claims. Dictionaries define a quack as "a pretender to knowledge." Thus a nutrition quack is a pretender to knowledge of nutrition.

Can you suggest some simple ways to recognize nutrition quackery?

Here is a list of twenty-two clues to quackery adapted from the writings of two of the country's leading "quackbusters": Victor Herbert, M.D., J.D., Chief of the Hematology and Nutrition Laboratory, Bronx V.A. Medical Center and Professor of Medicine at Mt. Sinai School of Medicine in New York City, and Stephen Barrett, M.D., coauthor of this book. You may want to copy this list for easy reference.

Clue #1: The Basic Sales Pitch. Beware of anyone who tells you all of the wonderful things that vitamins, minerals, and other nutrients do in your body, and what can happen if you don't get enough. This pitch neglects to tell you that nutrient deficiencies are rare; that if you are basically healthy, a balanced diet based on the Basic Four Food Groups will provide the nutrients you need; and that balancing your diet is simple.

Clue #2: The "Nutritionist" Hoax. Only a few states have laws defining the word "nutritionist" and restricting its use to individuals with recognized professional credentials. In the rest of the states, anyone can use this title whether qualified or not. Unqualified "nutritionists" often belong to organizations that have scientific-sounding names but espouse unproven nonscientific methods.

Clue #3: The-Diet-Causes-All-Ills-Myth. Although diet is a factor in the development of some diseases, most diseases are not caused by faulty diet. Steer clear of anyone who says they are.

Clue #4: The Poor-American-Diet Myth. The main forms of poor nourishment in America are undernourishment in the poverty-stricken and overnourishment resulting in overweight. Most Americans are not undernourished and are not in danger of developing nutrient deficiencies. But food quacks recommend that everybody take nutritional supplements, "health foods," or both.

Clue #5: The Poor-Soils Myth. Claims that soil depletion and the use of chemical fertilizers cause malnutrition are pitches to promote the sales of food supplements and "organic" foods by undermining public confidence in the American food supply.

Clue #6: The Overprocessed Foods Myth. Modern processing methods and storage do not remove all nutritive value from food. Although some processing methods lessen nutrient content slightly, other methods increase it. A balanced diet (which includes some fresh foods) will supply the nutrients needed by people in reasonably good health.

Clue #7: The "Stress-Vitamin" Ploy. Several major drug companies have advertised that under "stress," and in common diseases, your need for nutrients is increased. Such claims are misleading because no such need is likely to rise above that provided by a proper diet.

Clue #8: The "Chemical" Ploy. Food quacks suggest that you buy "natural" or "organically grown" foods to avoid being "poisoned" by food additives and preservatives. This is another scare tactic intended to make you distrust our major food producers. The American food supply is the safest and most nutritious the world has ever known!

Clue #9: The "Nutrition Insurance" Ploy. This scare tactic suggests that taking a daily vitamin or vitamin/mineral supplement is the best way to be sure you are meeting your nutrient needs. The fact is that most Americans who take supplements don't need them. Moreover, there is more to good nutrition than vitamins and minerals. The best course of action for people worried about the adequacy of their diet is to keep a diet diary for a week or so and have it evaluated by a registered dietitian or other qualified professional.

Clue #10: The "More-Is-Better" Pitch. Food quacks encourage people to take more than the Recommended Dietary Allowances of many nutrients but rarely warn that excesses can be dangerous to health.

Clue #11: The "Something Extra" Ploy. The claim that "natural" vitamins are better than "synthetic" ones is a plain and simple lie. The body cannot tell the difference (although your wallet may detect one).

Clue #12: The Diet-Cures-All-Ills Myth. This is one of the quack's cruelest and most dangerous claims because it may persuade people to seek dietary "cures" instead of effective diagnosis and medical treatment. Food quacks promote a large and steadily increasing list of foods and "food supplements" with supposed curative properties.

Clue #13: The Anecdotes-Are-Proof Ploy. Lacking scientific evidence in the form of controlled scientific studies, quacks use testimonials and case histories to support their claims.

Clue #14: The Phony Vitamin Ploy. Because vitamins are so popular, quacks have dreamed up a few of their own. The most notorious phonies have been "B_{15}" (pangamate) and "B_{17}" (a designation used to promote the quack cancer remedy laetrile). Others include choline, para-aminobenzoic acid (PABA), inositol, and rutin, none of which has any nutritional value for humans.

Clue #15: The "Doctors-Are-Butchers" Ploy. Quacks make sweeping claims that surgery, x-rays or drugs cause more harm than good. This is another scare tactic designed to drive people away from proven methods and into the hands of the quacks.

Clue #16: The "Alternative" Ploy. Pseudoscientific practitioners like to portray their approaches as "alternatives" to orthodox medical care. While some offer to "detoxify" your body, others claim to "balance" its chemistry, bring it in harmony with nature, or "strengthen your immune system" with special diets and various supplements.

Clue #17: "The-Scientific-Community-Is-Out-To-Get-Me" Claim. Promoters of unproven methods typically claim that the medical community is afraid of their competition and is somehow conspiring against them with the help of the food industry and the government (chiefly the FDA). Keep in mind that doctors and their loved ones also get sick. Can you really believe that the medical community or anyone else would try to suppress an effective remedy?

Clue #18: *The "Controversy" Claim.* Quacks would like you to believe that their claims are the subject of controversy among scientists. (Controversy does exist between quack claims and scientific facts.) Be especially wary of anyone represented as "a scientist ahead of his time." More than likely, he is a quack who has never caught up with the times.

Clue #19: The "Magic Diet" Myth. Huge fortunes can be made by persuading the public that a particular diet (or pill or gadget) will erase pounds or inches quickly and easily. If any such method existed, do you think millions of people would still be struggling to reduce?

Clue #20: The "Sugar-Is-A-Poison" Myth. Beware of those who claim that table sugar causes a long list of serious diseases. It does not (see Chapter 10). Despite a history of bad press, sugar is completely safe in moderate amounts.

Clue #21: The "Shut-Up-Or-I'll-Sue-You" Gambit. Promoters of quackery are often legally belligerent toward their critics, threatening legal action—and on rare occasion, actually filing suit. One of us (F.J.S.) has been sued twice (unsuccessfully) and threatened with suit several other times.

Clue #22: The "Freedom-Of-Choice" Ploy. Many quackery promoters state that consumers should be free to obtain any health product or service they desire without government interference. What these promoters really want, however, is to abolish consumer protection laws so they can sell whatever they please.

Why is nutrition quackery so widespread?

Probably because it is so successful financially! Quackery is a lucrative business. Since everyone has to eat, the potential market for nutrition quacks is huge. A clever person can—despite lack of education in the field of nutrition—convince a multitude of even well educated people that he or she is a nutrition expert offering dependable dietary advice.

What makes people vulnerable to quackery?

Most people who are fooled are simply unsuspecting victims of cleverly orchestrated publicity. Modern food quacks play on people's fears and take advantage of their hopes. People who are ill, particularly those with incurable diseases or chronically painful or disabling conditions, often become desperate enough to try anything. In addition, some people have strong feelings of alienation toward scientific medicine (and technology in general) and prefer to use what they consider to be "natural" methods.

To what extent are medical doctors involved in quackery?

The public has a right to expect that professionals licensed to practice medicine will be rational and base their practice upon scientific principles. Unfortunately, several hundred medical and osteopathic physicians seem to have abandoned scientific thought, particularly about body chemistry. These doctors commonly refer to themselves as "nutritionally oriented," "metabolic," or "holistic" physicians.

What's wrong with "holistic medicine"?

The term "holistic" is used in both orthodox (scientific) and unorthodox circles. However, considerable confusion surrounds its use. Orthodox practitioners regard holistic medicine as treatment of the "whole patient," with due attention to emotional factors as well as the patient's lifestyle. But others who label their approach "holistic" use a variety of unscientific methods of diagnosis and treatment. Competent physicians have always tried to understand their patients as whole beings, but the "holistic movement" is being promoted as something new by unscientific practitioners and crusading laypersons.

Chiropractors have been particularly active in organizing "holistic" and "wellness" centers that offer natural "treatments and preventive" services. The methods they recommend usually include spinal "adjustments" and unnecessary food supplements. Other bizarre methods used by unorthodox "holistic" practitioners include iridology (described below), acupressure, reflexology (a method based on the belief that pressure on the hands or feet can cure most diseases), and "applied kinesiology" (a treatment system based on the belief that muscle imbalance, correctable by massage and food supplements, is a major cause of disease).

In contrast, "wellness" programs run by scientific practitioners stress attention to "risk factors." These programs offer help in stopping smoking, provide counseling to promote weight control and a balanced diet, and teach exercise methods that improve cardio-vascular health and endurance.

Wallace I. Sampson, M.D., Clinical Professor of Medicine at Stanford University School of Medicine, calls the holistic label "a banner around which all manner of questionable practitioners are rallying." In *The Health Robbers* he recommends that scientific practitioners abandon the word "holistic" and its associated slogans because "the concept has been irretrievably corrupted by confused practitioners and promoters of quackery." We agree.

What is "chelation therapy"?

A number of "nutritionally oriented" doctors claim that intravenous administration of disodium EDTA (ethylenediamine tetra-acetic acid) plus various vitamins, amino acids, and other substances can cure serious diseases. Advocates of this method—which they call "chelation therapy"—claim that their injections clean the bloodstream of undesirable mineral deposits in order to cure heart disease, arthritis, multiple sclerosis, Parkinson's disease, kidney disorders and many other illnesses. The typical program includes twenty to fifty injections that cost $50 to $75 each.

Disodium EDTA, a chelating agent, has legitimate use in the treatment of lead poisoning and related conditions. When injected intravenously, it can bind lead or other metallic poisons to speed up their excretion from the body. Disodium EDTA is also used as a food preservative. However, no well designed tests have demonstrated that intravenous use is effective against any disease, and some cases have been reported in which chelation therapy actually caused kidney damage and death. A controlled trial whose protocol was approved by the FDA is now underway to test whether chelation therapy is effective against intermittent claudication, a condition in which impaired circulation to the legs causes pain when the person walks. Critics of chelation therapy believe that no benefit will be found. But even if benefit is found, this would not prove that chelation therapy is effective against heart disease.

What is "clinical ecology"?

"Clinical ecology" is based on the notion that multiple symptoms are triggered by hypersensitivity to common foods and chemicals.

Advocates of this belief describe themselves as "ecologically oriented" and consider their patients to be suffering from "environmental or ecological illness," "cerebral allergy," "total allergy syndrome," or "twentieth century disease," which can mimic almost any other illness.

Clinical ecologists claim that hypersensitivity to common substances develops when the total load of physical and psychological stresses exceeds what a person can tolerate. To diagnose "ecologically related" disease, practitioners perform various nonstandard tests, the main one being "provocation and neutralization." In this test, the patient reports symptoms that develop after various concentrations of suspected substances are administered under the tongue or injected into the skin. If any symptoms occur within ten minutes, the test is considered positive and lower concentrations are given until a dose is found that "neutralizes" the symptoms.

Treatment involves avoidance of suspected substances and lifestyle changes that can range from minor to extensive. Patients are usually instructed to modify their diet and to avoid such substances as scented shampoos, aftershave products, deodorants, cigarette smoke, automobile exhaust fumes, and clothing, furniture, and carpets that contain synthetic materials. Extreme restrictions can involve staying at home for months or avoiding physical contact with family members. In many cases, the patient's life becomes centered around the prescribed treatment.

The American Academy of Allergy and Immunology, the nation's largest professional organization of allergists, considers clinical ecology "speculative and unproven"—which is a polite way of saying that it is nonsense. Last year, researchers at the University of California issued a devastating report suggesting that clinical ecology is based entirely on placebo responses. Eighteen patients who had been diagnosed as allergic by experienced clinical ecologists were given provocation and neutralization tests by their own doctors using a double-blind protocol approved by clinical ecology proponents. No difference was found between the symptoms following food extract injections and those that followed injections of dilute salt water.

What is homeopathy?

It is a system of treatment that uses a wide variety of herbs, drugs, and other chemicals in infinitesimal doses. It is based on the theory that, if a substance can produce symptoms of illness in healthy persons, a tiny amount of the substance can cure the illness in a sick person. Homeopathy enjoyed some success during the nineteenth century when its methods (the equivalent of doing nothing) were less dangerous than some of the orthodox treatments of that period. Its remedies should still be regarded as placebos.

What is naturopathy?

Naturopathy is an elaborate pseudoscience based on the concept that the basic cause of disease is a violation of "natural laws." Naturopaths claim to remove the underlying causes of disease and to stimulate the body's natural healing processes. Naturopathic treatment methods include "natural food" diets, vitamins, herbs, tissue minerals, cell salts, manipulation, massage, diathermy, colonic enemas, acupuncture, reflexology, and homeopathy. Some practitioners of naturopathy are chiropractors; others are graduates of schools of naturopathy. A few states license graduates of naturo- pathic schools as independent practitioners. Many chiropractors and naturopaths believe that their methods are appropriate for the treatment of almost all diseases and conditions.

I've heard claims that a hair sample can be used to evaluate the body's nutritional status. Is that true?

No. A few practitioners—including self-proclaimed "nutritionists," some chiropractors, and a few other licensed professionals—claim that hair analysis is a valuable clinical tool. For about $40, they will send a sample of your hair to a laboratory for analysis of its mineral content. Most of the laboratories doing commercial hair analysis issue computerized charts of "excesses," "deficiencies," and/or "imbalances," with recommendations for correcting them with vitamins and other supplements, which typically are sold by the practitioner.

Despite claims made by the entrepreneurs who recommend hair analysis, your hair is not an accurate reflection of the adequacy of your diet. Hair does not contain any vitamins, and scientists have not determined what levels of minerals in hair should be considered "normal." Moreover, the mineral content of hair is readily influenced by non-dietary factors in the environment such as shampoos and conditioners, hair sprays, bleaches and dyes, and even air and water pollutants. At the present time, hair analysis can only provide trained scientists with limited information to assist in the diagnosis of heavy metal poisoning. Unlike a valid dietary analysis completed by a registered dietitian, a hair analysis will not help you to improve your diet, and it could lead you to upset your health as well as your budget.

What sort of nutrition training do chiropractors have?

Although chiropractors are licensed as "doctors," their scientific training is usually quite minimal. Chiropractic is based on the false theory that most diseases stem from spinal problems. Chiropractors' advice often includes nutrition "tips" that are scientifically unfounded and a threat to budget and/or health. Many chiropractors sell vitamins in their offices—for two to three times what they pay for them. Some also sell oral enzymes, "glandular extracts," homeopathic remedies, and similar quack products described in Chapter 5. Several companies marketing primarily through chiropractors sponsor seminars in which chiropractors are taught how to use supplement concoctions to treat virtually anything. For example, one such product—composed of ten vitamins, six minerals, three amino acids, RNA (from yeast), and "raw brain concentrate"—is touted for "nerve support," memory, alcoholism, and mental disorders.

How useful are computers for determining the nutritional composition of recipes or menus?

During the past decade the number of available nutrition programs has grown markedly. There are now more than a hundred software packages designed for microcomputers. These programs range in content and complexity from simple ones for schoolchildren to comprehensive models used by research scientists. Not all of these programs are accurate, and the wide choice can make it difficult to select the best one.

Many registered dietitians have been trained to use computers for diet planning and have access to computers programmed to do just that. If you require a special diet, you may ask a dietitian to analyze your current food intake, recommend any necessary changes, and provide you with menu plans and recipes. If you prefer to analyze your own menus, be sure to select a software package that suits your needs. You may want to preview the program or consult a dietitian before purchasing a software package for home use. The U.S.

Department of Agriculture, which has a software preview center at its National Agricultural Library in Beltsville, Maryland, has published a review collection called the "Food and Nutrition Information Center Software List."

Is it practical for consumers to use a home computer program for nutritional self-analysis?

Research indicates that many people have difficulty comprehending nutrient analysis of food products and drawing accurate conclusions. It is important for home users to recognize that computer data are based on food composition tables and have some limitations. Like food tables, computer data on the nutrient value of specific foods are approximations.

Programs suitable for home use that are reliable and are updated regularly to include new data on nutrient values and new food products include:

• "Eat Smart," for Apple computers, covers 136 food items and 12 nutrients [$19.95 from Pillsbury Co., Pillsbury Center, Minneapolis, MN 55402].

• "You Are What You Eat," for IBM or Apple hardware, covers 1,000 food items and 13 nutrients [$79.95 from DDA Software, P.O. Box 26, Hamburg, NJ 07419].

• "DINE," for IBM or Apple hardware, covers 3,400 food items and 15 nutrients [$190 from DINE Systems, 2211 Main St., Building B, Buffalo, NY 14214].

What about questionnaires used to tell whether someone needs to take vitamins or other supplements. Are these legitimate?

Those we have seen were sales gimmicks, designed so that almost everyone tested is found to "need" supplements. One, for example, was the "Vitamin Gap Test," promoted widely by the Council for Responsible Nutrition (CRN), a trade association of supplement manufacturers. CRN's test was so narrowly worded that many people with well balanced diets would be advised that they have possible "gaps."

A more elaborate gimmick was the "Nutritional Fitness Profile," a 29-question test offered by Great Earth Vitamin Stores, the nation's second largest health food store chain. Great Earth advertised that it would use the results to "tailor a nutrition support program [of supplements] that's a perfect fit for you." The questions pertained to diet, illnesses, lifestyle factors, and various symptoms that have little or nothing to do with nutrient deficiency. Neither the individual questions nor the test as a whole provided a legitimate basis for prescribing supplements.

A questionnaire based on the Basic Four Food Groups could be used to help determine whether someone's diet contains adequate amounts of nutrients. However, if a real problem is found, the best solution is likely to be dietary change rather than supplementation.

I've seen computerized dietary analyses offered in "health food" stores and by direct mail. Are they reliable?

Most, if not all, are schemes to boost the sales of food supplements. Computerized analyses offered directly to the public without benefit of professional interpretation seem to be programmed to tell everyone that supplements are needed. Some schemes involve completing a questionnaire that is scored by a computer. Others involve entering the data into the computer yourself and getting advice on the screen or in a printout.

Who can give reliable nutrition advice?

For medical advice, see a reliable physician. If you want dietary counseling, a registered dietitian or other nutritional professional would be more appropriate. Legitimate nutritionists are college graduates, usually with a master's degree and/or training in dietetics, who can provide reliable information about weight control, diet, and health. Some nutritionists have a doctoral degree as well. Nutritionists serve as educators in schools and universities, conduct workshops for community groups, or work in clinics or hospitals. Many nutritionists have a private practice through which they offer nutrition counseling to individuals and groups. They also collaborate with physicians and consult for hospitals and various companies.

If you want to lose weight safely and effectively, if your physician has diagnosed a diet-related illness such as diabetes, or if you have some general questions about nutrition and health, then a registered dietitian can probably help you.

How can I locate a reliable nutritionist?

Ask your doctor to refer you to one who practices privately or at a local hospital outpatient clinic; or contact your local hospital directly. The practitioner may require a written referral from a physician, since your medical history, your current medical problems, and your physician's dietary recommendations are important. Some private practitioners advertise in local newspapers or in the Yellow Pages under "Dietitian" or "Nutritionist," but check carefully before selecting someone from the Yellow Pages, because in most states phone companies don't attempt to screen out individuals who lack credentials. A list of registered dietitians in private practice in your area can be obtained by sending a self-addressed stamped envelope to Consulting Nutritionists, 9212 Delphi Road, S.W., Olympia, WA 98502.

Fees for private nutrition counseling vary according to geographic location, type of counseling (individual is more costly than group), and length of counseling sessions. Note, however, that a competent nutritionist will not prescribe or sell expensive supplements or suggest costly "superfoods." Instead, you will be taught how to balance your diet to suit your own individual needs, and how to select the foods you need from your local supermarket.

Reliable advice may also be obtained from a nutrition extension agent at any land-grant university or from a home economist at a USDA County Cooperative Extension Service office. Your telephone book can tell you whether your community has either of these services available.

How can I judge an individual's credentials?

Professional nutritionists have documented educational backgrounds in the field of nutrition from reputable institutions. Most have a master's or doctoral degree in nutrition from an accredited university. Registered dietitians (R.D.s) have had formal training in nutrition for at least four years, completed an approved special training program or its equivalent, passed a registration examination, and have been approved by the American Dietetic Association (ADA), the largest national organization of nutrition professionals. To remain registered, the R.D. must meet the ADA's requirements for continuing education in nutrition on a regular basis.

Nutritionists with doctoral degrees (M.D. or Ph.D.) can become certified by the American Board of Nutrition. Membership in the American Institute of Nutrition or the American Society for Clinical Nutrition is also a sign of reliability in the field. These organizations have strict requirements and do not admit promoters of nutrition quackery as members.

How can I tell if someone's credentials are dubious?

Unfortunately, the number of inadequately trained individuals who call themselves "nutritionists," "nutrition consultants," or "nutrition counselors" has grown rapidly during the past few years. Several questionable schools and a variety of other organizations have issued certificates that may look impressive but are based on little or no training in the science of nutrition and, in some cases, on mere payment of a fee.

One such school was Donsbach University, of Huntington Beach, California, whose president, Kurt Donsbach, was a former "health food" store operator and a chiropractor by background. Donsbach University, primarily a correspondence school, issued "B.S.," "M.S.," and "Ph.D." degrees in nutrition based upon the study of theories and practices contrary to those of the scientific community. Some Donsbach University graduates administer a computerized "Nutrition Deficiency Test," which leads to recommendations of large numbers of unnecessary food supplements. Some graduates practice "iridology," a system of diagnosis based on the far-fetched theory that inspection of the eyes can divulge a wide range of ailments curable with nutrition supplements. Donsbach University also issued a variety of other certificates based on shorter courses of study. For example, health food retailers who completed a $495 course on the "true facts" of nutrition received a "Dietary Consultant" certificate to display in their store. Donsbach University was sold and renamed International University for Nutrition Education in 1987 but is no longer in operation.

Bernadean University, another California-based "school," issued mail-order diplomas based on even less "training." One of us (V.A.) secured a "Nutritionist" degree for $84 even though she deliberately attempted to fail the course. On the first "test," Virginia answered the 35 true-false questions in accordance with nutrition facts. Since nearly one-third of her answers contradicted information given in the school's lessons, she expected to get a grade of 70 or below. However, the test was returned with a grade of 90, with a letter from the "office administrator" stating: "You may use the book for answers as it is an open book course. I just seem to feel that you put the answers in the wrong column." On the second test, Virginia answered all of the short-answer questions accurately so that her grade—based on information given in the course—should have been a zero. Yet she received a grade of 100% and an accompanying note congratulating her on the "excellent manner in which you have completed the Nutrition course." The "Nutritionist" certificate, obtained for an additional $10, contains an attractive gold seal and indicates that she graduated "Cum Laude"!

Schools like the above can be distinguished by the fact that they are not accredited by an accreditation agency recognized by the U.S. Secretary of Education or the Council on Postsecondary Accreditation (1 Dupont Circle, N.W., Washington, DC 20036). Schools accredited through recognized agencies teach reliable nutrition concepts—with two notable exceptions. Despite the fact that chiropractic and naturopathic schools teach unscientific methods, they do have accrediting agencies approved by the U.S. Secretary of Education. Some chiropractic schools can even issue an accredited degree in "clinical nutrition."

Checking credentials sounds like it could be complicated. Is there a simpler way to tell whether an individual is engaged in unscientific nutrition practices?

The simplest way is probably to avoid anyone who sells vitamins or states that everyone needs to take them.

How can I tell whether an organization promotes questionable nutrition methods?

You should be able to tell by examining the theories expressed by its members and publications. The main point is not to be impressed merely because an organization has a scientific-sounding name. Some of the organizations involved in the spread of questionable nutrition are:

American Academy of Environmental Medicine
American Association of Nutritional Consultants
American College of Advancement in Medicine
American Holistic Medical Association
American Natural Hygiene Society

American Nutritional Consultants Association
American Nutritional Medical Association
American Nutritionists Association
American Quack Association
Cancer Control Society
Committee for Freedom of Choice in Medicine
Confederation of Health Organizations
Council for Responsible Nutrition
Foundation for the Advancement of Innovative Medicine
Huxley Institute for Biosocial Research
International Academy of Nutrition and Preventive Medicine
International Association of Cancer Victors and Friends
International Association of Dentists and Physicians.
Life Extension Foundation (of Hollywood, Florida)
National Health Federation
National Nutritional Foods Association
Nutrition for Optimal Health Association
Orthomolecular Medical Society
People's Medical Society
Price-Pottenger Nutrition Foundation
Project Cure
World Research Foundation

What organizations do you recommend?

The following groups—all nonprofit—offer reliable publications and advice on nutrition. The ones marked with an asterisk (*) operate information clearinghouses about quackery:

*American Council on Science and Health, 1995 Broadway, New York, NY 10023

American Dietetic Association, 216 W. Jackson Blvd., Chicago, IL 60606

American Institute of Nutrition, 9650 Rockville Pike, Bethesda, MD 20014

American Medical Association Department of Personal Health, 535 N. Dearborn St., Chicago, IL 60610

American Society for Clinical Nutrition, 9650 Rockville Pike, Bethesda, MD 20014

Council for Agricultural Science and Technology, 137 Lynn Ave., Ames, IA 50010

Institute of Food Technologists, 221 N. LaSalle St., Chicago, IL 60601

International Life Sciences Institute—Nutrition Foundation, 1126 16th St., N.W., Washington, DC 20006
   *National Council Against Health Fraud, P.O. Box 1276, Loma Linda, CA 92354
   U.S. Department of Agriculture Food and Nutrition Information Center, Room 304, 10301 Baltimore Blvd., Beltsville, MD 20705
   U.S. Food and Drug Administration, 5600 Fishers Lane, Rockville, MD 20857.
   Accredited colleges and medical schools with nutrition departments may serve as excellent sources of information, as can state and local health departments.

What do you think of the quality of nutrition information available in newspapers and magazines?

It varies a great deal. While some journalists are quite reliable, others are not. Nutrition advice in the tabloids is especially untrustworthy. Dr. Stephen Barrett, who evaluated nutrition articles over a 13-week period during 1987, judged the percentage of accurate articles to be: *Sun* (38%), *Globe* (32%), *National Enquirer* (25%), and *National Examiner* (22%).
   As far as magazines are concerned, you should be suspicious of any "health" magazine that carries a great deal of advertising for dietary supplements. Such magazines usually boost unnecessary supplements in their articles as well. As far as general interest magazines are concerned, the American Council on Science and Health (ACSH) periodically evaluates nutrition articles published by twenty-five popular magazines. Table 3:1 summarizes ACSH's 1988 evaluation. Appendix C includes the names of several magazines and newsletters that offer reliable nutrition advice on a regular basis.

Table 3:1. Nutrition coverage in 25 major magazines.

Magazine	Rating	Comments
Excellent		
Consumer Reports	90	Aggressively fights misrepresentation and myths with thoughtful scientific analysis
Saturday Evening Post	80	Thoughtful analysis, sometimes too technical

Magazine	Rating	Comments
Good		
Vogue	79	Well balanced, accurate articles
Redbook	76	Serious and factual articles
Reader's Digest	74	Could better utilize other sources
Parents	74	Good mix of professionally written articles
Good Housekeeping	73	Covers a wide spectrum of topics with good sources
Changing Times	72	Consistently reliable stories and good sources
Women's Day	71	Presents reliable, practical advice
Modern Maturity	71	Relatively accurate and well presented
Seventeen	71	Reporting could be more complete
McCall's	70	Generally good, noncontroversial coverage
Fair		
Better Homes & Gardens	69	Fair, noncontroversial reporting
Glamour	69	Limited in-depth coverage of topics
Self	68	Some reliance on sensational reporting
Prevention	68	Large improvement seen, but still overemphasizes supplements
American Health	67	Objective reporting that is intelligent and practical
Health	67	Educational and informative, but overemphasizes supplements
Consumers Digest	66	Tendency toward advocacy—promoting one food or nutritional theory
Essence	64	Needs more scientific sources
Mademoiselle	62	Needs to expand nutrition sources
Family Circle	61	Effective at discussing issues in lay terms
Cosmopolitan	61	Makes some exaggerated claims. Heavy emphasis on slimming
Poor		
Gentlemen's Quarterly	58	Inconsistent treatment of topics, focusing on fads. Needs more sound information
Ladies Home Journal	52	Over-reliance on anecdotes and generalities

**Can you comment further on the quality of the
advice offered in "health food" stores?**

In 1983, three researchers from the American Council on Science and
Health reported the results of 105 inquires made at "health food"
stores in New York, New Jersey and Connecticut. Asked about eye
symptoms characteristic of glaucoma, seventeen out of twenty-four
suggested a wide variety of products without even seeing the
sufferer; none recognized that urgent medical care was needed.
Asked by telephone about a sudden unexplained fifteen-pound
weight loss in one month's time, nine out of seventeen recommended
products sold in their store; only seven suggested medical evaluation.
Seven out of ten stores carried "starch blockers" (a weight-loss
fraud) despite an FDA ban. Nine out of ten recommended bone meal
and dolomite, products that often are hazardous due to contamination
with lead. Nine stores contacted made false claims of effectiveness
for bee pollen and ten stores did so for RNA (discussed in Chapter
5). The study concluded that most "health food" stores give out
irrational, unsafe, and illegal advice.

In 1989, volunteers for the Consumer Health Education Council
telephoned forty-one Houston-area health food stores and asked to
speak with the person who provided nutritional advice. The callers
explained that they had a brother with AIDS who was seeking an
effective alternative against the HIV virus. The caller also explained
that the brother's wife was still having sex with her husband and was
seeking products that would reduce or eliminate her risk of being
infected. All forty-one retailers offered products they said could
benefit the brother's immune system, improve the woman's
immunity, and protect her against harm from the HIV virus. Thirty
said they sold products that would cure AIDS. None said, "Use a
condom or don't have sex."

**If "health food" stores give unsound advice
and are breaking the law, why don't law
enforcement agencies try to stop them?**

The violations involved are under the jurisdiction of state and local
authorities. A few retailers have been successfully prosecuted in
California for practicing medicine without a license, but as far as we
know, no other prosecutions have taken place. State medical boards
and local district attorneys seem apathetic for three reasons: 1)
prosecution of cases of this type requires considerable effort,

including undercover investigation; 2) since few "health food" customers realize they are being misled, enforcement agencies get few complaints; and 3) agency officials tend to feel that victims of nutrition quackery "should know better" and deserve what they get. Florida and California recently passed laws making it illegal for retailers to recommend products as effective against a long list of diseases and conditions.

How much protection against misleading "nutrition" practices does the federal government provide for consumers?

Not enough! Although the Federal Trade Commission (FTC) has jurisdiction over misleading advertising, it files only a few complaints each year against companies making misleading claims for foods or food supplements. The FTC's address is Sixth & Pennsylvania Ave., N.W., Washington, DC 20580.

The FDA has jurisdiction over product labeling. Although many "remedies" promoted as "food supplements" are misbranded, the agency has not been forceful enough in policing this area. The FDA's address is 5600 Fishers Lane, Rockville, MD 20857.

The Postal Service, which has jurisdiction over products sold by mail, enforces mail fraud laws vigorously, but most misbranded food supplements are not sold by mail. The Postal Service's address is 475 L'Enfant Plaza, Washington, DC 20260.

More vigorous enforcement by the FTC and FDA would be very helpful in protecting the public against certain types of nutrition quackery. But no government agency can protect consumers against false ideas promoted through broadcasts and publications, which are protected by freedom of speech and of the press.

What should I do if I encounter a misleading advertising message or questionable "nutrition" treatment of the type described in this chapter?

Most authorities would advise you to complain about false advertising to the appropriate federal agency. However, asking your Congressional representative to forward your complaint to the appropriate agency is likely to be more effective in the long run. It is important that elected officials realize that their constituents want protection, and it is important that federal agencies receive reassurance that Congress supports such protection.

Another agency that is sometimes effective against false advertising is the National Advertising Division (NAD), Council of Better Business Bureaus, 845 3rd Avenue, New York, NY 10022. During the past few years, NAD has exerted pressure against a few large companies that used misleading scare tactics to promote the sale of vitamins. However, its track record is inconsistent. Its vice president thinks most people should take vitamins for "insurance" and can see nothing wrong with the "Vitamin Gap Test" mentioned earlier in this chapter.

If you encounter a questionable practice performed by a licensed health professional, complaints should be filed with the individual's local or state professional society (if he or she is a member) and the state licensing board. If a questionable practitioner is not licensed, the state board should be asked to investigate whether he or she is practicing medicine without a license. If you feel you have been seriously damaged by a quack, the National Council Against Health Fraud's Task Force on Victim Redress can advise you about how to proceed.

Nutrition faddism and quackery are deeply rooted in our society. Health professionals can provide the facts. But only you can use them to protect yourself from being harmed.

4

Vitamin and Mineral Supplements

"If some is good, then more must be better." Such is the philosophy of those who advocate large doses of vitamins for an endless list of ailments. The public appears quite vulnerable: surveys have found that large percentages of American adults think that extra vitamins increase "pep" and energy and generally lead to improved health. That simply is untrue.

Minerals, too, have become the subject of quack promotions. Although some segments of our population are truly at risk for certain mineral deficiencies, supplementation is rational only when prescribed on the basis of demonstrated need.

What harm can excessive amounts of vitamins cause?

When scientists speak of excessive amounts of nutrients, they mean amounts that exceed the Recommended Dietary Allowances (see Chapter 1). While small excesses are harmless, large ones may cause trouble.

Prolonged intake of high dosages of vitamin A can cause a long list of adverse effects, including loss of appetite and hair, extreme drying and thickening of the skin, serious eye problems, increased brain pressure (mimicking a brain tumor), and abnormal bone growth.

Vitamin C in megadoses is dangerous and can cause gout and kidney stones in predisposed individuals. People taking high dosages for many months who stop too suddenly may suffer from bleeding gums, painful joints, and other symptoms of "rebound scurvy." Megadosage of vitamin C can also cause diarrhea.

Prolonged excessive intake of vitamin D can cause lack of appetite, nausea, headache, fatigue, kidney damage, calcifying of tissues, high blood pressure, and elevated blood cholesterol.

Excessive intakes of vitamin E can cause headaches, extreme fatigue, muscular weakness, nausea, diarrhea, blurred vision, skin rash, increased bleeding tendencies, and—contrary to what promoters of the "sex vitamin" would have you believe—reduced sexual function.

B-vitamins in large amounts can also produce adverse reactions. Large doses of niacin, for example, may cause flushing, itching, irregular heartbeat, elevated levels of blood glucose, gout, and serious liver damage. Excess folic acid can mask an otherwise discoverable deficiency of vitamin B_{12} that causes permanent damage to the nervous system. Excessive doses of B_6 can also be toxic to the nervous system, causing numbness and tingling of the hands, difficulty in walking, and electric shocks shooting down the spine— symptoms resembling those of multiple sclerosis.

Supplement promoters rarely warn against the dangers of vitamin megadosage.

Do healthy young adults need to take vitamin supplements to ensure good health?

Few people actually need to take vitamin supplements. As noted in Chapter 2, a varied diet composed of foods selected from the Basic Four Food Groups will provide adequate amounts of not only all the vitamins, but of other required nutrients as well.

Vitamins can be useful in the treatment of certain diseases and in recovery from surgery, burns, and serious illnesses where food intake is inadequate. But for healthy individuals, the best way to ensure optimal nutrition is to eat properly. If you are healthy and eating a balanced diet, all the vitamins you need will be available from your food—far more pleasantly and much less expensively than from a pill bottle.

What about the elderly? Should they take supplements for "insurance"?

Generally no. Like young adults, elderly individuals consuming a balanced diet based on the Basic Four Food Groups will receive adequate amounts of all nutrients. The elderly are usually less active physically, so have lower calorie needs, making it important that they select mostly nutrient-rich foods. Supplements may be appropriate for elderly individuals whose nutritional status is threatened by poor appetite and/or inadequate absorption, but these should be prescribed by their physician based on real needs rather than for "nutrition insurance."

Are vitamin supplements needed to cope with stress?

No! Several major pharmaceutical companies have advertised widely that "stress can rob you of vitamins." Others have suggested that vitamins should be taken to prevent "vitamin burnout" or "stress burnout" (conditions as yet undiscovered by modern science). The ads suggest that cigarette smoking, common respiratory infections, moderate use of alcohol and over-the-counter drugs, and even athletic activities will increase vitamin needs to the point that supplements should be taken to ensure an adequate supply. The truth is that such common stresses cause only insignificant increases in nutrient needs—which are easily met by a well balanced diet. So-called "stress supplements"—which contain high doses of vitamin C and B-vitamins—are a waste of money.

The concept of stress supplements was strongly attacked in the March 1986 issue of *Consumer Reports* magazine in an article called "The Vitamin Pushers." In it, the chief nutritionist for Lederle Laboratories (makers of *Stresstabs*) acknowledged that "People who eat a balanced diet do not need stress vitamins—or for that matter, any vitamins at all." Later that year, after the New York Attorney General objected to ads touting *Stresstabs* "for people who burn the candle at both ends," Lederle paid $25,000 to New York State and agreed not to represent that emotional stress causes vitamin depletion or that *Stresstabs* will reduce the effect of psychological stress. In 1990, the Federal Trade Commission and three state attorneys general forced Miles Laboratories, makers of One-A-Day brand supplements, to stop making unsubstantiated claims that its products are necessary or useful for replacing vitamins or minerals lost through physical exercise or the stress of daily living.

Are B-vitamins effective against mental illness?

During the 1950s a handful of psychiatrists began adding massive doses of niacin to their treatment of schizophrenia and other severe mental problems, an approach they called "megavitamin therapy." Now called "orthomolecular therapy," this approach has been expanded to include other vitamins, minerals, hormones, and diets, which may be used alone or combined with standard treatments. Experts who have reviewed the claims of megavitamin/ortho-molecular proponents have concluded that they are unsupported by scientific evidence.

My 2-year-old son refuses to eat any vegetables. Should I give him a daily vitamin supplement just in case?

Not necessarily. Fruits, dairy products, meats, fish, breads, and cereals are all good sources of vitamins, so if his overall diet is reasonably varied, his vitamin intake will still be adequate. Vegetables do serve to improve the variety and texture of the diet and are excellent sources of certain vitamins as well as fiber. However, the strong flavor of many vegetables makes them unpopular with young children. You might experiment with such tasty and nutritious dishes such as zucchini bread and spinach lasagna, which disguise their vegetable flavor. Tomato sauce is another vegetable item that many children like. So ignore any urges to nag and simply set a good example by eating a variety of vegetables yourself. Most children eventually learn to like vegetables when allowed to explore new tastes at their own pace.

Can vitamin A prevent cancer?

Vitamin A occurs in two major forms. Preformed vitamin A is primarily retinol, while provitamin A, which the body converts to vitamin A, is mostly beta-carotene. Preformed vitamin A is found only in foods of animal origin. Liver is an especially rich source, and whole milk, eggs, butter, most cheeses, and fortified margarines also provide preformed vitamin A. Carotene is a plant product abundant in deep orange and dark green leafy vegetables and fruits such as carrots, sweet potatoes, pumpkin, squash, dandelion, mustard and collard greens, spinach, broccoli, cantaloupe, peaches, and apricots.

Several researchers have reported that synthetic forms of vitamin A may have anticancer activity in animals, but it is not known whether these results are relevant to humans. Epidemiological studies indicate that some populations with above-average blood levels of vitamin A have a decreased incidence of certain cancers. But many factors other than vitamin A intake could be responsible for the decreased incidence of cancer. Studies are being conducted to see whether carotene and some synthetic forms of vitamin A can protect humans against certain forms of cancer.

**Would it be prudent to take vitamin A
supplements in case this nutrient is
ever proven to prevent cancer?**

No. Excess amounts of vitamin A are stored in body fat and can build up to toxic levels over long periods of time. Carotene is not as dangerous, but excessive intakes can produce carotenemia, a condition in which the skin turns orange. It does not make sense to take supplements of vitamin A or anything else unless strong evidence indicates that the benefits outweigh the risks.

Is vitamin C effective against the common cold?

Vitamin C has been investigated for possible value in preventing infections ever since it became commercially available during the 1930s. At least sixteen well designed, double-blind studies have found no preventive effect. In these studies, neither the experimental subjects nor the researchers knew which subjects were given vitamin C and which received a placebo. A few studies suggest that a modest excess of vitamin C may reduce the symptoms of a cold, but the effects are slight at best. Linus Pauling's belief that megadoses of vitamin C can prevent colds is based on his analysis of the same information considered by other scientists, but his conclusions are different. The vast majority of experts in the fields of medicine and infectious diseases disagree with him.

Is vitamin C effective against cancer?

No relationship of this sort has been proven. Consuming a diet that emphasizes fruits and vegetables may be associated with reduced risk for certain cancers. However, it is not clear whether this is related to the vitamins in these foods, other nutrients that are present, the amount of fiber, the fact that such diets tend to have less fat and fewer calories, and/or a host of other factors, both dietary and nondietary.

Linus Pauling also touts his favorite vitamin for the treatment of cancer. However, neither independent analysis of Pauling's data nor three large-scale studies at the Mayo Clinic and elsewhere support his claim that megadosage of vitamin C is effective as a treatment for cancer.

Are the "natural" vitamin C preparations made from rose hips or acerola berries more powerful than synthetic supplements?

The total vitamin content of a supplement product is provided on its label. If the vitamin comes from a "high potency" source such as rose hips or acerola berries, the potency is still no more than the number of milligrams stated on the label. Actually, supplements represented as vitamin C from rose hips or acerola berries usually contain only a small percent of the total amount of this vitamin from the "natural" source. The remainder is synthetic vitamin C, added to bring the total amount up to that stated on the label.

There is no need to resort to supplements, "natural" or synthetic, to get the small amount of vitamin C your body needs. A glass of orange or grapefruit juice, a wedge of cantaloupe, a tomato, or a serving of broccoli or Brussels sprouts will provide the recommended dietary allowance plus other nutrients as well.

Is vitamin E effective against breast lumps?

Several years ago, a preliminary study by a research team in Baltimore suggested that vitamin E supplements might help women with fibrocystic breast disease. But subsequent studies that were larger and conducted with a double-blind protocol found no beneficial effect.

**My husband insists on taking a vitamin E
supplement every day—or night!—because he
thinks it helps his sex life. I keep telling
him that only I can do that! Am I right?**

We can't answer your question in full, but your husband is certainly
wrong in assuming that vitamin E supplements aid sexual vigor. In
fact, excessive intake of this vitamin may have the opposite effect.
The myth that vitamin E helps virility arose from the misinterpretation
of experiments which showed that female rats (not male rats)
deficient in vitamin E have decreased fertility (not virility). Vitamin E
is so plentiful in the foods we eat (vegetable oils, whole grains, and
leafy vegetables, for example) that deficiency caused by faulty diet
has never been reported in humans.

**Should physically active adults take
iron supplements for extra energy?**

Iron, like all minerals (and vitamins), does not provide calories and
thus cannot serve as a source of energy. Iron-deficiency anemia will
result in general fatigue, but the presence of this disorder should be
determined by blood tests, and its treatment should depend upon the
cause. In men, for example, iron-deficiency anemia is often a sign of
internal bleeding.

Extra iron is required only when the body has to manufacture
more red blood cells than usual. This occurs after blood loss and
during periods of growth. Women who menstruate lose blood
monthly. Pregnant women, infants, and growing children also
require extra iron. Most people can get the iron they require by
including iron-rich foods in their diet. Liver, other meats, dark green
leafy vegetables, whole grain or enriched breads and cereals, dried
fruits, and legumes are all good sources of iron.

**Are mineral supplements needed to replace what
is lost through food processing or home cooking?**

A well balanced and varied diet—including fresh, commercially
processed, and home-cooked foods—can provide ample amounts of
all the minerals essential to good health. Moreover, it is safer to meet
nutrient needs by eating a wide variety of foods than by taking
supplements.

In excessive dosages, minerals can have toxic effects, especially the trace minerals required only in very small amounts. Selenium, for example, is toxic in amounts not much above the trace amounts needed. Large doses of zinc, another popular supplement, can cause nausea, vomiting, and irritability.

Food is obviously the most sensible source of minerals in the amounts the body needs. And although the less processed foods—dairy products, meat, vegetables (including frozen vegetables), and whole grains—tend to be richer in mineral content, convenience foods, fast-food fare, and other processed products also add to daily mineral intake.

The only exceptions to the no-need-to-supplement rule are the minerals iron, fluoride, and calcium. Iron is difficult to absorb, except from meats, so that individuals who require extra iron—pregnant women and women of childbearing age—may need to take a supplement. Vegetarians may also develop iron deficiency, since meat is one of the best sources of this mineral, and their typically high fiber intake can reduce iron absorption. The need for iron supplementation should be determined by a physician.

When are fluoride supplements advisable?

Fluoride is an essential mineral nutrient that helps to form strong teeth and bones, thereby contributing to a reduced incidence of dental decay and possibly to prevention of osteoporosis. Fluoride is usually low in the diet unless one lives in a community where the water supply is fluoridated. The American Academy of Pediatrics and the American Dental Association recommend that children in non-fluoridated communities take daily supplements as follows:

Table 4:1. Supplemental Fluoride Dosage

Age (years)	Concentration of fluoride in water (parts per million)		
	0.0 to 0.3	0.3 to 0.7	Over 0.7
Birth to 2	0.25 mg	none	none
2 to 3	0.50 mg	0.25 mg	none
3 to 12	1.00 mg	0.50 mg	none

When are calcium supplements appropriate?

Postmenopausal women are prone to develop osteoporosis, a condition characterized by brittle, porous bones. This disease is responsible for many back problems and bone fractures from minor falls. A generous supply of calcium is an important part of the prevention and treatment of this condition, but it is not the only factor involved. Cigarette smoking and lack of exercise also are risk factors.

Adequate amounts of calcium can be provided by three to four servings of milk daily—preferably using low-fat or skim-milk products—or by other milk-based foods. Other sources of calcium are less efficiently absorbed. Women who are unable to consume milk products should consult a physician or registered dietitian for advice on calcium supplementation. Once osteoporosis has developed, self-treatment with calcium supplements is unlikely to be much benefit. Hormones are usually required as well, which requires close medical supervision.

Is there any chance of obtaining too many vitamins or minerals by eating fortified foods such as breakfast cereals?

It is unlikely but, like anything else, fortified foods should be eaten in moderate amounts. The real potential danger from eating too much fortified food is caloric excess and the accompanying problem of overweight.

Is there now too much iodide available in the food supply?

Not long ago, individuals living in certain areas of the U.S. with iodide-deficient soils were prone to develop thyroid gland enlargement (goiter) due to iodide deficiency. With the iodization of salt, this disorder has become rare. In recent years, use of iodide-containing dough conditioners by the baking industry has increased the iodide content of the American diet to a point where scientists have cautioned against further increases. But there is no reason to worry about current levels.

Can zinc supplements help my diminished sense of taste?

Unless your diet is unbalanced, it is unlikely that your problem is due to a zinc deficiency. Animal foods, especially meat and eggs, are good sources of this nutrient. If, like most Americans, you are consuming adequate amounts of protein, you are probably receiving enough zinc as well. High-fiber diets can cause some zinc losses, but unless you are a strict vegetarian following a diet that includes excessive fiber, the decrease in the sensitivity of your taste buds is probably not due to a lack of zinc. Supplements should only be taken if prescribed by your physician after a deficiency has been diagnosed. Zinc toxicity can cause kidney failure, anemia, muscle incoordination, and other dangerous side effects.

Perhaps your diet is dull rather than your sense of taste. Instead of wasting your money on zinc supplements, why not try out some new foods and seasonings? Oysters Rockefeller, a Spanish omelet, and broiled chicken tarragon are enticing sources of both zinc and good taste.

My doctor has prescribed a diuretic that can deplete potassium. Do I need to replace my losses with a potassium supplement?

Potassium supplements should not be taken unless prescribed by a physician. Including some potassium-rich foods in your diet can help to protect you from deficiency, but if a deficiency does develop, potassium supplements will probably be necessary. Potassium-rich foods are listed in Table 4:2.

Certain conditions decrease the body's ability to excrete excess potassium. Such a disorder and/or misuse of potassium supplements can lead to the potentially fatal condition of hyperkalemia (excess potassium in the blood). Unrestricted use of salt substitutes containing potassium can also cause undesirably high intakes of this mineral. Thus, the Food and Drug Administration advises consumers to use potassium supplements and potassium-containing salt substitutes only under the supervision of a physician. A glass of orange juice or a banana in the morning and a serving of broccoli or avocado with lunch or dinner are safer and much tastier ways to provide an adequate potassium intake.

Table 4:2. Potassium-rich Foods

Food	Portion Size	Potassium (mg)
Fruits		
Grapefruit juice	1 cup	420
Orange juice	1 cup	500
Prune juice	1 cup	600
Tomato juice, low-sodium	1 cup	550
Apricots, dried	10	345
Avocado	1/2	680
Banana	1 med.	440
Cantaloupe	1/2	680
Dates	10	520
Prunes	10	450
Raisins	1/2 cup	550
Vegetables, cooked		
Broccoli	1/2 cup	205
Cauliflower	1/2 cup	130
Potato (with skin)	1 med.	555
Spinach	1/2 cup	290
Squash, winter	1/2 cup	475
Sweet potato	1 lg.	340
Meat and dairy products		
Chicken, light meat	3 oz.	370
Eggs	2 lg.	130
Ground beef, lean	3 oz.	220
Milk, whole	1 cup	350
Milk, skim	1 cup	355
Pork, lean	3 oz.	280
Steak, lean sirloin	3 oz.	305
Tuna (in water)	3 oz.	235
Grains and legumes		
Lentils, cooked	1/2 cup	250
Oatmeal, cooked	1 cup	145
Peanuts, in shell	20	250

Can selenium supplements prevent cancer?

Selenium is an essential trace mineral that, like vitamin E, functions in the body as an antioxidant. The claims for cancer-preventing ability stem from this property, but evidence so far does not support use of this mineral for preventive or curative purposes for any type of cancer. Seafood, whole-grain cereals, meats, and eggs can be good sources of selenium. Illness due to dietary deficiency of selenium has never been reported in this country.

Like other minerals, an excessive intake of selenium is undesirable, and oversupplementation can result in harmful side effects. Another important danger associated with self-prescribed mineral supplements may be the failure to attain necessary medical care. Save your money and your health—adopt a health-promoting lifestyle, don't use tobacco products, and be wary of sensational and unproven dietary cancer "cures."

Are silicon and boron essential nutrients?

Silicon is now known to be an essential trace mineral for certain animals, but no proof exists that it is essential for humans. Research is underway to explore a possible relationship between silicon and the aging process and between boron and the prevention of osteoporosis. Someday, silicon and boron may be recognized as essential trace minerals for humans. In any case, there is no need to be concerned about developing a deficiency of either one as long as your diet is well balanced and varied. Instead, it is important to understand that excessive intakes may have toxic side effects.

Are bone meal supplements dangerous?

They certainly can be dangerous. Heavy metals such as lead are stored in bones. The amount stored depends on the lead content of the food and water consumed by the animals whose bones are ground to make the bone meal. Commercial bone meal is usually prepared from the bones of old cattle or horses, and the lead (or other heavy metal) content may be dangerously high.

A serious example of the toxic effects of bone meal was reported several years ago in the *Journal of the American Medical Association.* A 46-year-old actress was hospitalized in southern California with a diagnosis of lead poisoning. She had been taking one to two ounces of powdered bone meal daily for several years. Several other cases of lead poisoning in people taking bone meal supplements have been reported since then.

Is it sensible for lactating mothers to take dolomite to obtain extra calcium?

It is unwise for breastfeeding mothers to self-prescribe supplements of any kind. They can obtain all the calcium necessary by including three or more servings from the Milk and Cheese Group in their daily diet. For those unable to tolerate milk products, a safe calcium supplement can be prescribed by the attending physician. Dolomite, however, can be dangerous because some preparations have been found to contain unhealthy levels of toxic minerals such as arsenic and lead, as well as certain other contaminants.

Remember, food is nature's own packaging for the nutrients most people require for proper growth and health.

5

"Health Foods" and Other Magic Potions

There have always been food fads and fad foods. Dr. William Jarvis, professor of public health and preventive medicine at Loma Linda University, notes that throughout history there have been four major types of "magic potions": the fountain of youth, the love potion, the cure-all, and the athletic superpill. Most of today's potions are "food supplements" and "health foods" promoted through publications, broadcasts, and claims made by retail salespeople. Some of these products have even made their way into special "nutrition centers" in supermarkets and pharmacies.

Modern-day nutrition quacks are well aware of the vulnerabilities of their potential victims. They are expert at playing on public fears and can sound quite scientific to those who lack the background to evaluate their claims.

**Can you estimate the
cost of nutrition quackery?**

Exact figures do not exist. But it is clear that the costs of unnecessary vitamins, overpriced "health foods," unproven "nutrition" remedies, and weight-reduction scams amount to billions of dollars a year in the United States alone—and even more when you consider how much some victims pay in suffering, false hope, and delay of effective medical treatment.

Can you define the term "health food"?

The term "health food" is merely a gimmick used to boost sales. Food faddists use it for any food that supposedly makes a special contribution to health. The nutrients in foods can be determined by scientific analysis. Some foods marketed as "health foods" are rich in nutrients, but no food has unique health-promoting properties. All foods can contribute to good health when eaten as part of a varied and balanced diet. The problem with so-called "health foods" is that they are promoted with false claims and usually are overpriced.

What is a food supplement?

In common usage, the term refers to any food substance or mixture of such substances consumed in addition to, or in place of, food. The most commonly used food supplements are vitamins and minerals These, of course, are essential nutrients. Some products sold as supplements (such as lecithin, PABA, and bioflavonoids) are *not* essential because they contain nothing the body needs or cannot make itself. Some products (such as Laetrile, Gerovital, and B$_{15}$) that are neither essential nor ordinarily found in the diet are marketed as "food supplements" with the hope of avoiding prosecution for illegal drug claims.

Here, in alphabetical order, is a catalog of current "food supplements" and "health foods." Those marked with an asterisk (*) deserve special attention. Some cause health problems when taken in large amounts, while others pose direct health risks, even in moderate amounts.

Acidophilus

Lactobacillus acidophilus is a bacterial organism that can ferment the sugars present in milk and milk products such as yogurt. Acidophilus supplements are claimed to aid digestion and improve the health of the digestive tract. This is impractical, however, because the bacteria in oral doses may not be alive or may fail to survive the acidic environment of the stomach. Yogurt, kefir, and other fermented milk products are nutritious but offer no proven curative benefit.

For individuals who have difficulty digesting lactose—a condition called "lactose intolerance"—certain preparations (such as Lact-Aid) can be of practical value. These products contain lactase, an enzyme that helps to digest the lactose in milk. However, if you are lactose-intolerant, it is advisable to obtain guidance from a physician.

Activated charcoal

Supplements labeled "activated organic charcoal" are usually made from "natural organic peat moss." They are promoted as agents that will absorb intestinal gases and "serve as a powerful detoxicant" to combat "gas" and "make you feel intestinally clean." Actually, this supplement is ineffective and can even add to gastrointestinal distress by interfering with the action of some digestive enzymes. People troubled by "gas" should learn to eat more slowly so that they swallow less air. They should also avoid any foods that tend to cause problems for them. Common culprits are carbonated beverages (including beer), chewing gum, apple peels, and gas-forming fruits and vegetables such as melon, dried fruits, onions, cabbage, and beans.

Alfalfa*

Although advocates of this plant suggest that it offers certain nutrients that more common plant foods do not, alfalfa actually has less nutritional value than most of the more popular vegetables such as broccoli, carrots, and spinach. Claims have been made that alfalfa contains all of the essential amino acids, but this is also untrue. Some advocates of alfalfa supplements and extracts promise the additional benefits of "antitoxin properties" and the ability to "prevent exhaustion." There is no scientific evidence to support these claims. Alfalfa tea, a popular herbal tea, contains saponins, which can adversely affect digestion and respiration.

Aloe vera*

Despite the many claims made by proponents of this plant, aloe juice has never been shown to be an effective remedy for arthritis or any other health problem. Using aloe creams and gels on your skin is probably harmless. Even though it won't reverse the inevitable process of aging, topical aloe may produce some skin softening and moisturizing effects. However, aloe juice taken internally acts as a laxative and can cause gastrointestinal upset.

If you like rubbing aloe-containing creams onto your skin, by all means do so. But steer clear of using aloe as a food supplement, oral medicine, or menu item. Internally, the aloe plant is useless at best, and can even be dangerous.

Amino acids*

Various amino acid combinations have been marketed as "growth hormone releasers" that cause weight loss while you sleep. These claims are based on faulty extrapolation of animal experiments. Amino acid combinations are also marketed as "steroid substitutes" that can help build large muscles. This claim also is false.

L-tryptophan, an amino acid touted for sleeplessness, depression, premenstrual syndrome (PMS), and weight control, was recently implicated in an outbreak of eosinophilia-myalgia syndrome, a rare but serious disorder characterized by severe muscle and joint pain. More than 1,500 cases and several deaths were reported. The difficulty was due to a contaminant introduced during the manu-facturing of tryptophan by a Japanese supplier.

Bee pollen

Promoters of bee pollen claim it is a "perfect food" that contains a wide variety of nutrients. But it contains no nutrients that are not present in ordinary foods. Bee pollen is also touted as an aid to athletic performance. Actual tests on swimmers and runners have shown no benefit. At up to $45 per pound, bee pollen is ridiculously overpriced as a source of nutrients. Tell anyone who tries to convince you otherwise to "buzz off!"

Beta-carotene

Promotion of beta-carotene supplements boomed after the National Academy of Sciences published a report on diet, nutrition, and cancer in 1982. The NAS report did not recommend supplements but merely observed that populations whose intake of foods rich in beta-carotene (and other substances) is high may have a lower incidence of certain cancers. Beta-carotene is abundant in bright orange and dark green vegetables and certain fruits. It still is not known what substances (if any) in these foods exert a protective effect or whether the effect is due to fiber content, antioxidants, or other factors. Researchers from Harvard Medical School are conducting a large double-blind study to test whether beta-carotene supplements can protect against cancer, but their experiment has not yet been completed.

Bioflavonoids

Bioflavonoids are promoted as essential for good health and to strengthen resistance to colds and the flu. Scientific tests have shown these claims to be false. Bioflavonoids have never been found useful for the treatment of any human ailment. They are sometimes referred to as "vitamin P," but they are neither vitamins nor essential for humans.

Blackstrap molasses

This product is the dark, less refined form of molasses. It is less sweet than other syrups and has a distinctive flavor. It is often touted as a "wonder food" that can restore hair color, cure anemia, and provide superenergy and a vast array of nutrients. Actually, it is simply a form of sugar. It does contain enough iron that consuming a few tablespoons of molasses at regular intervals can contribute significantly to the iron intake of anemia-prone individuals such as young women and the elderly. However, blackstrap molasses cannot reverse the graying process of the hair or produce other wondrous effects claimed by its proponents.

Bone meal*

Powdered bone is advertised as a rich source of calcium. Actually, calcium from bone meal is poorly absorbed. More significantly, many bone meal samples have been found to contain high levels of lead (a toxic mineral). Thus, bone meal supplements are not helpful and can be dangerous.

Bran*

Wheat bran is composed mainly of cellulose, an insoluble fiber that absorbs water and helps prevent constipation. Oat bran, which contains soluble fiber, can help reduce blood cholesterol levels. Rice bran may also have a cholesterol-lowering effect.

Moderate amounts of fiber-containing foods (whole grains, fruits, and vegetables) are a desirable part of a balanced diet. However, excessive amounts can cause bloating, cramps, diarrhea, and can interfere with the absorption of certain minerals. Significant cholesterol reduction cannot be achieved merely by adding a bit of bran to one's daily diet; it requires a comprehensive program of dietary and lifestyle changes—which is most likely to be successful if done under professional guidance. This topic is discussed further in Chapter 13.

Brewers' yeast

Brewers' yeast is the yeast used to ferment carbohydrate in making beer. It is a good source of protein and several of the B-vitamins, but it is no miracle food. If you actually enjoy the taste of brewers' yeast, you can add it to baked goods, mixed dishes, and hot cereal. But if you are like most people, who dislike its bitter taste, don't worry that you are missing out on any special nutritional value. A well balanced diet without brewers' yeast will supply all of the nutrients your body needs for good health. People with gout should avoid yeast.

Carob

Carob beans are legumes that have been cultivated in the Mediterranean area since ancient times. Sometimes called St. John's bread, carob has been used in dog biscuits, as a flavoring agent in chewing tobacco, and, more recently, as a chocolate substitute. Carob is lower in fat than chocolate and is caffeine-free, but it does not taste like the real chocolate that chocolate-lovers adore. Claims that carob has special health-promoting properties are false.

Chelated minerals*

"Chelate" means "to bind." Minerals in chelated supplements are usually bound to protein, which is claimed to enhance their absorption into the body. However, there is no scientific evidence to support this claim. Mineral supplements should not be taken unless prescribed by a physician. Individuals with a medically diagnosed need for mineral supplements can get adequate amounts from non-chelated forms, which are less expensive.

Chlorophyll

Chlorophyll is the pigment responsible for the green color of plants and enables them to trap energy from sunlight. Claims have been made that chlorophyll can cure or help cure a long list of health problems. All such claims are unfounded.

Choline

Not essential in the diets of humans, this compound is widespread in foods. Thus, even if we did require a dietary source, supplements would be unnecessary. Scientists are investigating the possible use of choline compounds in the treatment of certain brain disorders, but supplements will not improve memory or "counter the aging process," as claimed by supplement promoters.

Cider vinegar

Vinegar made from apples has long been recommended as a cure-all when taken together with honey, and sometimes with other food supplements as well. It is claimed to keep the body "in balance," thin the blood, and aid digestion—none of which is true. Cider vinegar is an acceptable condiment, but the myths surrounding its use should be ignored.

"Cold pressed" oils

Vegetable oils are relatively high in unsaturated fats (except for coconut and palm oil, which are high in saturated fats) and are good sources of vitamin E. Processing increases the safety of vegetable oils. Most oils are filtered to remove impurities, including odorous chemicals, and antioxidant preservatives are usually added to prevent development of rancidity. "Cold pressed" oils sold in "health food" stores undergo a different type of processing. Two types of these oils are available under various brand names: crude, which is dark and still contains sediment and plant solids; and the lighter, filtered version. Neither has any health advantage over oils processed by traditional methods. According to *Consumer Reports,* cold pressing takes place at anywhere between 140°F and 475°F—which is certainly not "cold."

Promoters of "cold pressed" oils often claim that regular vegetable oils don't contain vitamin E. Although refined oils may contain a bit less than the unrefined products, the difference is negligible. All vegetable oils are good sources of vitamin E—whether sold at reasonable cost, or "cold pressed" and sold at higher prices.

Desiccated liver

Liver is a very nutritious food, and the dehydrated form is also a rich source of many nutrients. But there is really no need for a healthy individual to rely on food supplements. If you eat a well balanced diet that includes a wide variety of foods selected from the Basic Four Food Groups, there is no need to purchase extra nutrients—at extra cost. An occasional serving of broiled chicken livers or liver and onions can provide all the nutrients found in the less tasty desiccated form, and for a reasonable price as well.

Dolomite*

Dolomite is mined from rocks and contains the minerals calcium and magnesium. However, these minerals are poorly absorbed from dolomite supplements and are often accompanied by large amounts of toxic metals. Lead, arsenic, mercury, and other contaminants have been found in dolomite samples in amounts that can damage health. Milk and milk products are more sensible sources of calcium; and legumes, green leafy vegetables, potatoes, and whole grains can supply all the magnesium we need for good health.

Enzymes (oral)

Enzymes are proteins that act as catalysts in the body, speeding up certain chemical reactions, such as those involved in the digestive process. All the enzymes required to digest food and catalyze other metabolic processes are produced within the body. The enzymes in food (or supplement concoctions) are digested in the body like any other protein: they are broken down to their component amino acids and don't enter the circulatory system intact. So don't be misled by claims that oral enzymes can "strengthen" your body's vital organs.

There is a minor exception to the above facts. Oral pancreatic enzymes given in enteric-coated capsules have a legitimate medical use in diseases that involve decreased secretion of pancreatic enzymes into the intestine. These diseases are not appropriate for self-diagnosis or self-treatment. Anyone who actually has a pancreatic enzyme deficiency may have a serious underlying disease that should be medically diagnosed and treated.

"Ergogenic aids"

Many concoctions of vitamins, minerals, and/or amino acids are marketed with false claims that they can increase stamina and endurance and help build stronger muscles. Ads for these products typically contain an endorsement from a champion athlete or bodybuilder who attributes success to the products. Some are touted as "natural steroids" or "growth hormone releasers," which they are not.

Evening primrose oil

Extracts from the evening primrose flower have been promoted in the health-food press as effective against premenstrual syndrome, rheumatoid arthritis, atopic eczema, and various other conditions. The largest producer of the oil is Efamol Ltd., a British company that has sponsored many research projects. Although it is possible that evening primrose oil (EPO) has valid medical uses, the company has not submitted evidence to the FDA that EPO is safe and effective for any such use. Instead, it promoted EPO in the United States as a "food supplement" that contains gamma-linolenic acid (GLA). At the same time, the company communicated through the media that various health problems are caused by a dietary deficiency of GLA— which the product can supposedly help. In 1988 the FDA seized large quantities of Efamol's EPO, charging that it was an "unsafe food additive" and also was being illegally marketed as a drug.

Fertilized eggs

Advocates of fertilized eggs may boast that fertilization by a rooster produces a health-promoting quality called "vitalism." But the eggs are actually nutritionally equivalent to their "non-vital" counterparts. And they tend to spoil faster and cost more.

Along similar lines, some food faddists claim that brown eggs are nutritionally superior to white eggs. This is untrue. Egg color is hereditary and has nothing to do with nutrient composition.

Fish oil capsules

Epidemiological research has found that Eskimos and others with diets rich in omega-3 fatty acids have less heart disease than Americans or Europeans. Other research has found that supplements of these fatty acids (found in fish oils) can help lower blood cholesterol levels and inhibit blood clotting, which means they may be useful in preventing atherosclerotic heart disease. However, it is not known what dosage is appropriate or whether long-range use is safe or effective for this purpose. The FDA has ordered about a hundred manufacturers to stop making claims that fish oil supplements are effective against various diseases, but it *is* legal to market the products without such claims. It is unwise to self-medicate with fish oil capsules. They should be used only by individuals at high risk for heart disease who are under close medical supervision. Eating fish once or twice a week may provide the benefits of fish oils without the risks.

Garlic

Raw garlic and garlic oil capsules are claimed to "purify the blood," reduce high blood pressure, and prevent cancer, heart disease, and a variety of other ailments. Some studies suggest that certain populations with large intakes of garlic exhibit a lower incidence of certain diseases, but further research is necessary to determine what factors are actually responsible. Until more evidence has accumulated, we suggest that you favor your good breath over the possibility that large amounts of garlic may one day prove to be a health aid.

Germanium

"Organic germanium" is touted as a "miracle drug" that is effective against everything from AIDS to zits. The main source of these claims appears to be the writings of Kazuhiko Asai (1908-1984), a Japanese metallurgist who theorized that cancer, heart disease, mental deficiency, and other problems are due to "oxygen deficiency within the body—which organic germanium can eradicate." There is no scientific evidence to support these claims.

A few germanium products have been tested for anti-tumor activity, but so far no practical applications have been found. Although many "health food" stores sell germanium products, it is illegal to market them with therapeutic claims. The FDA has banned importation of germanium products intended for human consumption and has seized germanium products from several U.S. manufacturers.

Gerovital H3 (GH3)

This substance is actually procaine, a local anesthetic better known as Novocain. Although claims have been made that Gerovital H3 is "the secret of eternal vigor and youth" and can cure everything from deafness to impotence, there exists no evidence to support such assertions. Nor is there good reason to believe that it can tighten wrinkles, repigment gray hair, or stimulate hair growth. Alas, we have yet to discover the fountain of youth!

Ginkgo biloba

The health food industry has been claiming that extracts made from the leaves of the ginkgo tree can "nourish brain cells," "reverse the aging process," and increase longevity. These claims are false. Ginkgo extracts may have the ability to increase cerebral blood flow, but there has not been sufficient research to settle whether they are useful for this purpose. Although gingko extracts are legally prescribed in certain European countries, they do not have FDA approval for sale as therapeutic agents in this country.

Ginseng*

Ginseng is a Chinese plant used for making herbal teas. Used for centuries, ginseng derives its name from the Chinese words for "man-plant" because the typical root resembles a human figure. Ginseng is promoted as a cure-all for illnesses ranging from impotence and stress to heart disease and cancer, as an ancient potion bearing "magical" powers, and as an edible fountain of youth for good health and long life. Claims are also made that use of this herb can provide a "joyful temper, plenty of pure red blood, relief for your irritable bladder," and increased sexual pleasure. Some ginseng roots sell for more than $300 per pound.

Unfortunately for naive consumers, ginseng has never been shown to provide any health benefit. In fact, excessive use of ginseng can produce a variety of problems—including elevated blood pressure, a dangerous side effect in individuals with hypertension. Other side effects include nervousness, insomnia, confusion, depression, and gastrointestinal disorders.

"Glandular extracts"

"Glandular extracts" sold as "food supplements" are claimed to cure diseases by augmenting glandular function within the body. Actually, they contain no hormones and thus exert no pharmacological effect on the body. If they did, of course, they would not be suitable products for self-treatment. Anyone with a hormonal problem should be under competent medical care.

Glutamic acid

Supplement salespersons are promoting a variety of concoctions to "increase memory power." One is glutamic acid, an amino acid manufactured within the body. Although scientists are studying the relationship between memory and the intake of certain amino acids, using supplements with the hope of improving brain function is certainly premature. Memory loss can be a sign of serious illness, particularly if it occurs before age 60, so a physician should certainly be consulted if this problem occurs. An unbalanced diet can cause nutritional deficiency that leads to memory impairment. If your diet is varied and reasonably well balanced, there is no reason to add amino acid supplements with the hope of improving your memory.

Goat milk

The milk of goats has been advertised as a more nutritious substitute for cow milk. Naturopath Paavo Airola, author of several books

promoting questionable nutrition practices, claimed that goat milk
contains special factors effective against arthritis and cancer. Goat
milk is no more nutritious than milk from cows. It is usually not
pasteurized and, like unpasteurized milk from any animal, it can carry
diseases in the raw state (see "raw milk," below). Airola, who
lectured widely on how to prevent aging, suffered a fatal stroke at the
age of 64.

Granola

Granola is the common term used to describe cereals and candy bars
composed largely of grains, fruits, seeds, and nuts. Promoted as
"natural" and rich in nutrients, granola products tend to be high in
sugar (usually brown sugar and/or honey), fats (from vegetable oils,
nuts, seeds, and coconut), and calories. A two-ounce serving of
cereal can contain over 250 calories. If you like the taste of granola
products and can afford the calories, go ahead and enjoy them. But
don't expect any health miracles—and remember that coconuts are
high in saturated fat.

Green-lipped mussel

Extracts of New Zealand green-lipped mussels have been promoted
as a treatment for arthritis even though there is no scientific evidence
to support this claim. To avoid prosecution for false labeling, the
product labels make no therapeutic claims. But such claims have been
promoted through magazine articles and a publicity tour by a British
author whose book tells all about these supposedly magical little
creatures. Several years ago the FDA banned importation of green-
lipped mussel extract and seized the supply of the leading American
distributor, but products can still be found on the shelves of some
"health food" stores.

GTF chromium*

GTF (glucose tolerance factor) chromium is derived from yeast that
has been grown in a chromium-rich medium or is isolated from pork
kidney. Health claims associated with this product include increases
in energy and stamina, improved cardiovascular fitness, and a
strengthened sense of overall well-being. Although chromium is an

essential nutrient, a varied diet provides an adequate supply. Glowing claims for GTF chromium supplements are highly exaggerated.

Gymnema sylvestre

Extracts of this herb are being marketed as a "sugar eliminator" and "sugar blocker," with claims that it prevents absorption of the sugar molecules found in food and therefore help in weight reduction and diabetes control. These claims are false. It has been known for more than a century that chewing the leaves of *Gymnema sylvestre* can prevent one from experiencing the sweetness of sugar. But there are no reliable studies showing that it can block the absorption of sugar into the body.

Herbs*

Many herbs are popular as flavoring agents for foods and as teas. Some are promoted as "natural" substances capable of preventing or curing diseases. To avoid trouble with the law, herbs sold through "health food" stores are labeled as flavoring agents or "food supplements." But pamphlets, magazines, and books make a wide variety of false claims that would be illegal on product labels.

It is beyond the scope of this book to examine the herbal market in detail, but a few basic points can be made. First, in the amounts typically consumed, herbs do not provide any significant nutritional contribution to the diet. Second, although a few herbs have healing properties (and some are the basis for modern drugs), few ailments that herbs are supposed to help are suitable for self-treatment. Third, certain herbs are potentially toxic. In a few cases, herbs have fatally poisoned unsuspecting consumers. Just because something is "natural" does not guarantee that it is safe to use. Some of the most toxic substances known are found in plants.

Incidentally, contrary to popular belief, some herbal teas contain caffeine. Read labels carefully or, if information is lacking, write to the manufacturer for a list of ingredients. If you drink herbal teas, make sure they are freshly brewed and that you drink only moderate amounts. Many substances are harmless in small doses but dangerous in large amounts. Avoid teas made from the herbs listed in Table 5:1. For more detailed information about herbs, read *The New Honest Herbal,* by Varro E. Tyler, Ph.D.

Table 5:1. Adverse Effects of Herbs

Herb	Problems
Chamomile (camomile), goldenrod, marigold, yarrow	Allergic reactions, including fatal allergic shock in persons sensitive to ragweed, asters, chrysanthemums and related plants
Buchu, quack grass, dandelion	Diuresis (loss of body water)
Catnip, juniper, hydrangea, jimson weed, lobelia, nutmeg, wormwood	Nervous system damage, hallucinations
Poke root	Nausea, vomiting, cramps, diarrhea
Burdock root	Atropine-like symptoms: blurred vision, dry mouth, hallucinations
Buckthorn bark, dock root, aloe leaves	Diarrhea
Senna (leaves, flowers, bark)	Cramps, diarrhea
Sassafras root bark	Contains safrole, a carcinogen (cancer-causing agent)
St. John's wort	Delayed allergic reactions, sun sensitivity
Pennyroyal, Indian tobacco, shavegrass (horsetail), mistletoe leaves, hemlock	Death
Ginseng, licorice	Increased blood pressure
Comfrey	Liver damage

Homeopathic remedies

Homeopathy (discussed in Chapter 3) is based on the notion that substances in extremely high dilutions can cause powerful effects by stimulating the body's "vital force." Some homeopathic manu-facturers advertise that their products "produce no side effects"— implying that they are superior to FDA-approved prescription and nonprescription drugs. Actually, most homeopathic remedies sold to the public are so dilute that they exert no pharmacological effect whatsoever. Although homeopathic remedies can be legally marketed within certain FDA guidelines, the agency has never required proof that they are effective.

Honey

Honey and table sugar have the same chemical make-up (fructose and glucose). Honey is crude sugar. It contains trace amounts of a few nutrients, not enough to make it significantly more nutritious than sugar. Honey provides such minuscule amounts of vitamins and minerals that you would have to eat a ridiculously large amount in order to derive any nutritional benefit. For example, to obtain the same amount of calcium contained in 1 cup of milk, you would have to consume 288 tablespoons of honey. Since honey is sticky, it can contribute to tooth decay. It is also more expensive than table sugar. The real differences between sugar and honey are taste and cost.

Inositol

Contrary to popular claims, supplements of inositol will not alleviate baldness, reduce blood cholesterol levels, or promote weight loss. Nor is inositol a B-vitamin—our bodies can manufacture all we need. Even if it were a vitamin, supplements would be unnecessary because it is readily available in our food supply. Recently, several health food store retailers announced that they stopped selling inositol powder because most of it was used to "cut" cocaine and methamphetamines.

Kelp*

Kelp is a seaweed common in the Japanese diet. Tablets of kelp are prepared from dried seaweed and promoted as a weight-reduction aid, a rich source of the mineral iodide, an energy booster, and a "natural" cure for goiter and several other certain ailments. Kelp is indeed high in iodide, a deficiency of which can lead to goiter. But iodized salt contributes plenty of this mineral to our diets, and at a fraction of the cost of kelp. Excess iodide can be detrimental to health and even lead to the development of a goiter.

Kelp is high in sodium, a mineral Americans tend to overconsume. Kelp is not a significant source of calories (hence energy), or of any other nutrients—aside from the two minerals mentioned—that are required by the body. The urine of some individuals taking kelp tablets has been found to contain elevated levels of arsenic.

Laetrile*

Laetrile is sometimes referred to as "vitamin B_{17}," but it is certainly not a vitamin! It is a trade name for amygdalin, a chemical found naturally in the pits of peaches, apricots, bitter almonds, and certain other plant materials. There is no scientific evidence that Laetrile inhibits the development or growth of cancer cells.

The so-called "evidence" presented by Laetrile supporters has consisted of testimonials given by various individuals who believe that Laetrile has cured them of cancer. One well known advocate of Laetrile was asked to submit files of his most dramatic cases of success to the Food and Drug Administration. Of the nine records reviewed, six patients had died of cancer, one still had cancer—which had spread since Laetrile had been taken—one had used approved drugs and radiation therapy, and one had died of another disease after having had the cancer surgically removed.

Laetrile is not harmless. It contains significant amounts of one of the most toxic substances known: cyanide. More important, many people have died as a result of using Laetrile instead of following proper medical treatment for cancer. But it is not difficult to sell hope to people who are desperate.

Lecithin

Despite claims by many proponents, lecithin has yet to be proven useful in the prevention or treatment of cardiovascular diseases—or anything else. The body manufactures its own supply of lecithin in the liver, and it is present in many foods as well, including soybeans, whole grains, and egg yolks. Contrary to faddist claims, lecithin tablets have not been shown to dissolve blood cholesterol or rid the blood stream of undesirable fats. Claims that lecithin supplements can cure arthritis, improve brain power, and aid in weight reduction are also unsupported by scientific evidence.

L-Lysine

Lysine, an essential amino acid, is promoted as a cure for herpes virus infections. Lysine's promoters claim that it prevents the virus from growing normally, that it can cause pain to disappear overnight, and that it can prevent the occurrence of new blisters. In 1982, acyclovir (marketed as Zovirax) received FDA approval for treatment of genital herpes. Acyclovir does not cure herpes, but it can shorten the duration of attacks and delay recurrences. At the present time, no evidence exists that any other substance, including lysine, can prevent or cure genital herpes. If you have this condition, or think you might have it, consult a physician.

Octacosanol

"Health food" advocates have claimed for many years that raw wheat germ contains an active ingredient they call "octacosanol," which they say has special benefits for athletes. This substance is present in many plant oils but is not essential in the human diet. Claims for improved stamina and endurance, blood cholesterol reduction, and reproductive benefits should simply be regarded as advertising hype. The Federal Trade Commission has forced a leading manufacturer to stop claiming that octacosanol can increase stamina and endurance. But such claims are still being made by others.

"Oral chelation" products

"Oral chelation" products composed of vitamins, amino acids, and various other ingredients are claimed to be effective in preventing or treating atherosclerosis. There is no scientific evidence that these products work. The FDA has ordered many manufacturers to stop marketing them, but a few are still available.

"Organically grown" foods

These are defined by their advocates as foods grown without the use of pesticides or manufactured fertilizer. But many studies have found little difference in pesticide content of foods labeled "organic" and those grown by conventional methods. Moreover, the miniscule amounts of pesticide residue in foods do not pose a threat to health. Nor does the type of fertilizer make much difference. Plants use the chemicals they need only in the inorganic state, so it matters little whether the plants are "fed" with manure, compost, or manufactured fertilizer. Without adequate nutrients, a plant will simply not grow. The soil serves mainly to support the plant. There is no rational basis for the belief that "organic" or "organically grown" foods are nutritionally superior to conventionally grown foods. Calling a certain food "organic" is like calling water "wet." Apples are apples; their vitamin content cannot be altered simply by changing the way they are grown. A food's vitamin content is genetically determined. Fertilizers may influence the content of a few minerals in plants, but this is rarely significant to the overall diet. "Organic" foods differ from conventional foods in only one respect: they usually cost much more. Unfortunately, a new federal law calling for the establishment of "organic" certification standards appears likely to generate more confusion.

Papain

Papain, an enzyme present in papaya extract, is promoted as a digestive aid, a cure for pyorrhea (gum disease), and a boon for weight reduction. As noted above, most enzymes taken by mouth are rapidly destroyed in the digestive tract, so they are unable to function as enzymes within the body. The only significant use for papain is as a meat tenderizer—added to meats before they are cooked.

PABA (para-aminobenzoic acid)

PABA is a vitamin for bacteria, not for humans. It is claimed to prevent or reverse the graying of hair, but no scientific evidence exists to support this claim. PABA is a useful ingredient in sunscreen lotions because it can help block the sun's ultraviolet rays. Oral intake of PABA won't do this.

"Passion flower" fruit

This berrylike fruit is sometimes used to flavor drinks and ices. It has been acclaimed as a folk remedy for everything from high blood pressure and pneumonia to insomnia and depression. This fruit contains a significant amount of vitamin C, but there is no evidence to support the cure-all claims.

Protein supplements*

Protein powders, tablets, and liquids are promoted as useful for building and strengthening muscles. These claims are false. It is quite easy to obtain all the protein your body requires with a well balanced diet. Meat, poultry, fish, eggs, milk, and cheese (as well as certain plant food combinations) can provide plenty of the protein essential for good health. Athletes usually obtain more than they need in the food they consume. Extra protein is not used to build muscles but is either burned for energy or stored as fat. As a sole food source, or in excessive amounts, protein supplements can cause nutritional imbalances, kidney ailments, and other health problems.

Raw milk*

Pasteurization is one of the important technological advances that have led to improved standards of health and safety for today's consumers. The unfounded fear that pasteurization destroys nutrients has led naive consumers to endanger their health by consuming "certified" milk or other types of raw (unpasteurized) milk. Although about 10 percent of the heat-sensitive vitamins (vitamin C and thiamin) are destroyed by pasteurization, milk would not be a significant source of these nutrients anyway. On the other hand, contaminated raw milk can be a source of harmful bacteria, such as those that cause undulant fever, dysentery, and tuberculosis. ("Certified" means that the cows have been proven free of tuberculosis, but it does not guarantee that the milk is free from other disease-producing organisms.) The FDA has banned interstate commerce in raw milk products, and a California Superior Court Judge has ordered the leading producer to stop advertising that its products are safe and healthier than pasteurized milk

RNA/DNA

Proponents of RNA and DNA supplements claim that these genetic materials can inhibit the aging process. Actually, when they are taken orally, they are broken down during digestion and inactivated.

Royal jelly

Royal jelly is food for queen bees. Claimed to increase endurance, it
has been recommended for athletes. It is also advertised as rich in
calcium pantothenate (falsely claimed to be "vitamin B_5,"), a
supposed antioxidant/antistress nutrient also used in "miracle" skin
creams and hair tonics. Royal jelly may be good for the queen bee,
but it is a ripoff for humans.

Rutin

Rutin, chemically related to the bioflavonoids, is not a vitamin and
has no known nutritional value for humans. It is illegal for
supplements to be labeled with nutritional claims for rutin, but it is
often added to multivitamins as "something extra."

Sea salt

Whether harvested from the sea or from mineral earth deposits, salt is
composed of sodium and chloride. Proponents of sea salt claim that it
is unrefined and therefore more nutritious, but it is actually refined to
remove impurities. Sea salt contains as much sodium as table salt,
but table salt can have the advantage of being iodized. "Seawater
concentrates" have been marketed with claims that they can cure
cancer, diabetes, and a whole host of other diseases. These claims
are both untrue and illegal.

Spirulina

Spirulina is an alga that forms a thick green scum on the surface of
fresh-water ponds and lakes. Several species of algae have been
harvested and marketed in capsules or tablets with claims that they
are useful in weight control and effective against allergies, visual
problems, anemia, and many other disorders. There is no scientific
evidence to support such claims, and a few manufacturers have been
forced to stop making them. Spirulina products—most notably blue-
green algae—are also said to be high in protein and rich in other
nutrients. However, the amounts contained in the commercially
marketed products are minuscule and can be obtained at much lower
cost from ordinary foods.

Sprouts

The nutritional value of sprouts is often exaggerated. Sprouted plants do contain modest amounts of vitamin C, but they do not contain a "life force," as enthusiasts have claimed. The sprouting process contributes the vitamin C lacking in the parent beans, but sprouts contain less of the other nutrients that dried beans provide.

Low in calories due to a high water content, sprouts can provide dieters with something relatively nutritious to chew on. They add bulk to sandwiches and salads, and provide various textures and flavors, depending on the type of bean from which they are sprouted. The nutrient content of the sprout depends largely on the parent bean.

If you enjoy eating sprouts, by all means do so. But don't fall for the romanticized health-promoting properties bestowed on this or any other "health food."

Superoxide dismutase (SOD)

SOD is an enzyme promoted as an "antioxidant" that supposedly protects body tissues against environmental contaminants and prevents heart disease, cancer, and arthritis. The body has its own supply of functioning antioxidants, including various enzymes and vitamins C and E. Enzymes taken orally are inactivated in the gastrointestinal tract. Thus, SOD supplements will not protect your body against smog, cigarette smoke, or anything else. The best strategy against air pollution is to live in an unpolluted environment and protest against polluters—including cigarette smokers. Donate your money to reputable causes instead of wasting it on unproven remedies such as SOD.

"Vitamin B_{15}"*

Like B_{17}, the substance called B_{15} is not a vitamin. It is also known as pangamate, pangamic acid, or Russian Formula. Its proponents claim it is effective against cancer, heart disease, alcoholism, diabetes, glaucoma, allergies, and schizophrenia. They also claim it can purify the air, provide the body with instant oxygen, and slow down the aging process. But there is no evidence that B_{15} has any therapeutic benefit or that it is safe to ingest. The FDA considers "vitamin B_{15}" a food additive for which no evidence of safety has been offered and has forced several manufacturers to stop selling it.

"Vitamin F"

Heralded as "a nutrient essential for your skin," so-called vitamin F is simply another name for essential fatty acids. Professional nutritionists don't use this term. Claims for "new vitamins," like those for "miracle nutrients," are simply advertising gimmicks.

Wheat germ

Wheat germ is a good source of protein, several B-vitamins, vitamin E, certain minerals, and fiber. But wheat germ is neither a miracle cure-all nor a dietary essential. It is provided amply in whole wheat products. If you enjoy the taste of wheat germ, feel free to sprinkle it on your cereal, or add it to casseroles and baked goods. However, ignore claims that it is a health-promoting superfood. As a supplement, it is relatively high in calories (from the fat in wheat germ oil)—and in cost.

Yogurt

Yogurt is nutritionally equivalent to the type of milk it is made from. It is a good source of calcium, riboflavin, protein, and other nutrients—as are all milk products—but it is certainly not a "perfect" food with magical anti-aging properties as is sometimes claimed.

***

Do the writings of Durk Pearson and Sandy Shaw contain valid recommendations for "anti-aging nutrients"?

In *Life Extension,* which catapulted Pearson and Shaw into the public spotlight several years ago, they suggest that animal experiments may now be adaptable for humans who wish to live to the age of 150—a suggestion with which the scientific community certainly disagrees. The book's introduction contains a two-page disclaimer, and cautions and warnings appear throughout the text in bold-face type. The authors' so-called "Current Personal Experimental Life Extension Formula" is a list of thirty-one food supplements and prescription drugs presented with a warning that it is "NOT RECOMMENDED FOR ANYONE OTHER THAN OURSELVES." Recommended instead is an extremely complex (and rather expensive) system of self-experimentation under close medical supervision that begins with more than fifty laboratory tests. We doubt that any sane doctor would participate in such a project.

The book's commercial success was due largely to hundreds of appearances by the authors on talk shows, especially the Merv Griffin Show. Later, Pearson and Shaw produced two more books and a videotape, began publishing a monthly newsletter filled with unproven supplement recommendations, and developed nutrition products marketed by several companies. They seem to have dropped out of the limelight, but their work has helped create today's large market for bogus "anti-aging products" and "ergogenic aids."

Are there any foods or nutrient products that can enhance immunity?

Although vitamin deficiency decreases immunity, there is no evidence that well nourished people can boost immunity by eating any special foods or by taking supplements. But public concern about AIDS (with its resultant focus on the immune system) has apparently inspired health food industry manufacturers to market a wide array of products that supposedly "strengthen the immune system."

Many health food stores carry products intended for the treatment of yeast infections. Are they legitimate?

No. A small number of health professionals have been promoting the bizarre notion that millions of Americans have a multiplicity of symptoms because they are hypersensitive to the common yeast *Candida albicans*. The American Academy of Allergy and Immunology considers this concept "speculative and unproven."

The most active promoter of "candidiasis hypersensitivity" is William G. Crook, M.D., author of *The Yeast Connection*. Many "health food" industry manufacturers paralleled his efforts by marketing "anti-candida" concoctions and "yeast-free" product lines. During the past two years, the FDA and FTC have curbed claims for several "anti-yeast" concoctions.

**Some "health food" enthusiasts recommend fasting
to purify the body and cleanse it of toxins.
Does this idea have any validity?**

There is no such thing as "purifying" the body. The concept is only a
meaningless expression for an old health fad. Fasting has not been
shown to contribute any benefit to overall health. Nor does lack of
food "cleanse" the body of "toxins." This is another old concept that
was probably religious in origin. In fact, ketones, the end products
of incomplete fat breakdown, which build up during the fasting state,
can be toxic. The dangerous side effects of prolonged fasting—
muscle and organ tissue breakdown, acid-base imbalance,
dehydration, fatigue, etc.—outweigh any possible psychological
benefit of "self-purification."

**Are "health foods" less fattening
than regular supermarket fare?**

Not usually. The only way to lose weight is to take in fewer calories
than you expend. This is best achieved by exercising more and eating
less—of everything, especially high-calorie, high-fat foods. Despite
claims to the contrary, "health foods" are neither more health-
promoting nor less caloric than comparable supermarket products that
usually cost much less.

Supposedly "healthier" alternatives to snack foods and desserts
are often advertised as appropriate for weight loss diets and marketed
through "health food" stores. Such items tempt naive dieters who
believe that "natural" foods are healthier and therefore can be
included without limit in a weight-loss diet. Sometimes the diet
claims are ambiguous, like the following message on a bag of "health
food" cookies: "You can eat as many of these tempting honey snaps
as you like—without guilt!" Yes, you can, if you don't feel guilty
about overeating cookies rich in butter, honey, and coconut, three
ingredients providing mostly calories with little nutritional value.
Carrot cakes, too, may seem like low-calorie treats. But they are
typically high in calories, loaded with sugar, coconut, nuts, and
vegetable oil, and topped with a high-fat frosting. A generous slice of
this rich dessert can contribute over 500 delicious calories!

Carob is another sneaky source of calories. Carob-flavored
brownies, cookies, candy bars, and other desserts usually have
caloric contents equivalent to their chocolate-flavored counterparts.

Obviously, the "health food" label is no guarantee that a product can promote health or assist with weight loss. Usually this tag merely indicates an inflated price.

If nutritious foods are good for your body, are they effective externally as well? I'm tempted to buy "organic" shampoos, "natural" cosmetics, and avocado, peach, apricot and other flavorful skin creams, all of which sound good enough to eat.

Purchase these products if they appeal to you, and if you find that their costs are justified by the results with your hair and skin. But you should realize that any nutrients available in these products will not be absorbed into your body, and they are unable to do much good when applied topically or washed into the scalp. You should also understand that any claims against the "synthetic chemicals" found in the less costly "unnatural" cosmetics are unfounded, since such products must be safety-tested and approved. Nearly all of the "natural" products also contain synthetically derived ingredients. Without preservatives, cosmetics would have to be kept under refrigeration and would last only a week or so.

Allergic reactions to cosmetics are not usually due to the "synthetic chemicals" but to the perfumes, many of which are derived from natural sources such as fruit oils and flower petals. "Hypoallergenic" cosmetics, on the other hand, do not have any added scents.

You can certainly use "natural" hair and skin products if you are satisfied with the results. Just don't expect any miracles. There is no product that can be applied to the body to stop the aging process.

Do you think it is fair to lump nutritious foods in the same discussion as quack cancer remedies?

This chapter discusses a wide variety of substances. Some are nutritious, some are not. Some are toxic per se, while others are dangerous only if used to excess. All have two things in common: they are promoted with false and misleading claims; they are often sold at high prices. If you like the taste of brewer's yeast, carob, granola, and wheat germ, and if you think that they are fairly priced, by all means enjoy them. But don't buy "health foods" because you think they are "magic potions." They are no more and no less nutritious than the nutrients they contain. They do not contain any special nutrients that cannot be found in a balanced diet. If you are inclined toward buying products promoted by the "health food" industry, familiarize yourself with the facts about them—particularly those that pose health hazards.

6

"Junk Foods" and "Fast Foods"

The term "junk food" is as meaningless as the term "health food." The dictionary defines "junk" as "useless stuff, trash, or rubbish," and describes "food" as "any substance taken into the body to maintain life and enable growth." Thus, "junk food" would be defined as useless stuff we take in to nourish ourselves—hardly a sensible combination of words!

Actually, all foods can be considered "health foods" in that they can contribute to good health when eaten as part of a balanced diet, and any food can become "junk" when so much of it is eaten that it crowds out the other foods necessary for a balanced diet. If you ate so much candy that your diet failed to include a variety of foods from the Basic Four Food Groups, your nutritional balance would be upset. But this would also hold true if you drank so much milk that you could eat little else: your diet would just as surely be unbalanced and deficient in important nutrients. Thus, any food can become a "junk food" if eaten to excess.

People who use the term "junk food" claim that we have a dismal dietary situation in this country and that all of us are filling up on nutritionless foods. But reputable nutrition surveys indicate that most Americans ingest much more protein than they need, and that the majority are meeting or exceeding most vitamin and mineral requirements. The most common nutrition problem in this country is not due to undernutrition but to overnutrition—that is, to excess calories from all kinds of foods and beverages.

The term "fast food" applies to the speed with which a food is prepared and served rather than the nature or content of the food itself. Actually, the term "fast-service food" might be more appropriate. There are now more than 55,000 fast-food restaurants throughout the United States. Fast foods are quick, convenient, affordable, and a popular component of the modern American lifestyle. The typical American now spends some $200 a year on fast foods, and the market is expanding.

Do so-called "junk foods" provide any nutrients, or do they only supply lots of calories?

Foods commonly thought of as "junk foods" include "fast foods" like hamburgers and pizza, snack foods like chips and soft drinks, and sweets like cookies or cakes. Although many of these foods are high in calories, the concept that these calories are "empty" or nutrient-free does not make sense. There is no such thing as an "empty calorie," since calories indicate that a food provides energy. Some so-called "junk foods," such as hamburgers and pizza, are quite high in nutrient value. In addition to the food energy (calories), many of these products provide carbohydrate, some contribute high-quality protein, and several offer significant amounts of vitamins and/or minerals as well. Look at the following nutritional analyses for two of our most popular "junk foods": ice cream and pizza. Nothing "empty" about these foods!

Table 6:1. Nutrient Content of Ice Cream and Pizza

Food and serving size	Calories	Protein (grams)	Carbohydrate (grams)	Other notable nutrients
Vanilla ice cream, 1 cup	260	6	28	Calcium Phosphorus Riboflavin
Pizza, 1/4 pie, 14" diameter	300	16	37	Calcium, Phosphorus Vitamin A Riboflavin

Note that ice cream is even richer in nutrients when it contains fruit and/or nuts, and vegetable-topped pizza can provide additional nutrients and fiber. Both of these foods also provide significant amounts of certain trace minerals. Many other popular "junk foods" contain nutritious ingredients. Consider the following examples:

    Pie: wheat flour, fruit, custard, nuts
    Cake: wheat flour, milk, eggs, sometimes fruit or nuts
    Hamburger: lean beef (bun has wheat flour, milk, eggs)
    Fried chicken: chicken, wheat flour, eggs
    Doughnuts: wheat flour, milk, eggs, sometimes fruit
    Cookies: wheat flour, milk, eggs, sometimes oats, nuts, or fruit
    Chips: potatoes or corn, vegetable oil
    Popcorn: corn, sometimes vegetable oil
    Milkshakes: milk, ice cream, sometimes nuts or fruit

These foods can add nutrients as well as pleasure to our diets.

Aren't fast foods likely to be low in vitamins and certain minerals?

Some fast foods are excellent sources of certain vitamins and minerals, while others are not. With wise selection, it is possible to maintain dietary balance even when some meals are purchased at fast-food outlets.

How can I select a nutritious meal at a fast-food restaurant?

Most fast-food restaurants offer a limited variety of foods but include salads, vegetables, fruit, and even low-fat vegetarian fare on their menu. With proper nutrition know-how, it's easy to fit the fast foods you enjoy into your total daily diet without upsetting your overall nutritional balance. A well balanced meal can be selected from almost any fast-food menu if the following concepts are kept in mind:

    • Choose a variety of different items. Avoid getting trapped in a "hamburger-and-cola" habit.

    • Limit your intake of fried foods, such as french fries, fried chicken, fried fish, sausage, and pepper steaks. Note that biscuits, donuts, croissants, and butter-soaked muffins are also high in fat.

    • Remember that some of the dessert choices contain considerable amounts of sugar and fat and have little other nutrient value.

    • Avoid salting your fast-food items since most already contain a significant amount of added salt.

• Select low-fat milk instead of whole milk, especially if you wish to decrease your caloric intake.

• Ask for lettuce, tomato, onion, green pepper, mushrooms, and other vegetables on sandwiches or pizza; use the salad bar where available, and limit dressings.

• Be sure that fast foods are only part of an overall well balanced diet.

Is it nutritionally unwise to lunch on submarine sandwiches?

An occasional submarine sandwich (sub, hoagie, grinder, hero, bomber, etc.) can certainly serve as a nutritious luncheon choice. Varying the fillings from day to day can provide needed variety. However, the typical sandwich of this size may pose a few problems worth considering:

Caloric content can be high.
Fat, cholesterol, and sodium (salt) content can be high.
Fiber content can be low.

Overweight individuals should be especially cautious about high-calorie choices. A twelve-inch sub roll alone contains close to 400 calories. Fatty, fried, mayonnaise-laden subs are high in calories because they are high in fat. Egg sandwiches are high in cholesterol, and cold cuts contain a considerable amount of salt. Pickles, pickled vegetables, and potato chips are also salty. Most subs are made with enriched rolls, which are nutritionally similar to whole grain breads except that they do not contribute much fiber to the diet.

Sub sandwiches can still be included in the diet, however, if selected wisely. The following tips may prove helpful when you next ponder over a submarine sandwich menu:

• Syrian bread is a low-calorie (230 calories per pocket) alternative to sub rolls. Some places offer whole wheat pockets.

• Half-size subs are often available.

• Turkey, lean roast beef, tuna, and chicken are all low-calorie, low-fat, low-cholesterol choices—but only if the subs are made with little or no mayonnaise.

• Vegetarian sandwiches offer more fiber and usually less fat.

• Request that lots of raw vegetables—lettuce, tomato, sprouts, peppers, mushrooms, onions, etc.—be included in your sub to increase both fiber and nutrient contents.

• Select milk to drink with your sub, preferably the skim or low-fat variety, or fruit juice.

Assuming that both breakfast and dinner are well balanced, a nutritious submarine sandwich can prove to be a tasty luncheon selection.

**I never have enough time for breakfast
on workdays unless I stop at a
fast-food outlet. Would it be better
to skip the morning meal altogether?**

No, don't skip breakfast. Almost everyone is aware that a good day begins with a good breakfast. Morning fatigue and lack of energy are more apt to afflict breakfast-skippers, and they tend to end the day with an insufficient total nutrient intake. Yet many busy consumers are skipping or skimping on this important meal.

Our typically fast-paced lifestyles have led to a large-scale shift away from the sit-down-family-style, bacon-and-eggs morning meal. Many people breakfast alone, consuming a bowl of ready-to-eat cereal, toast, coffee, and a glass of juice. If you don't care to eat breakfast at home, a quick stop at a fast-food outlet can provide you with a nutritious solution to your morning meal woes—as long as you make wise food choices.

Many fast-food breakfast selections are high in calories, fat, cholesterol, salt, and/or sugar. It is best to minimize your intake of fried foods, pastries, and fatty meats, and to limit your consumption of hash-brown potatoes, pancakes, waffles, croissants, Danish pastries, donuts, sausages, and bacon, as well as fried and scrambled eggs. Some preferable fast-food breakfast choices include:

• Muffins (corn, wheat bran, oat bran, or fruit)—though often higher in fat than the homemade kinds, these donut shop choices are usually the least caloric and lowest in fat. Note that large, heavy muffins may be significantly high in fat and calories.

• English muffins—request these without added butter, since the fast-food variety tend to come drenched with it.

• Dry cereals—select bran or whole-grain varieties, and request skim or low-fat milk.

• Fruit juice—sometimes fresh fruit is also available.

• Eggs—an occasional poached or boiled egg is a nutritious choice.

Some restaurants offer yogurt, buttermilk, cottage cheese, bagels, or whole-grain toast as well. As long as your lunch and supper meals are well balanced, a fast-food breakfast can certainly contribute to an overall healthy diet.

Should chronic waist-watchers avoid fast-food outlets like the plague?

Fast foods do tend to be higher in calories (and fat) than a lot of other meal and snack items are, but they certainly can be included as part of a well balanced diet. You can request nutrition information from your local fast-food outlets to determine the caloric and nutrient values of your favorite menu items. Remember, you can order small portions, choose regular burgers over giant-size specials, and request that items be prepared plain, unbuttered, and unsauced. Some fast-food outlets aim to accommodate dieters by offering "light" versions of standard fare, including leaner burgers, salads with low-fat dressing, and low-fat or nonfat frozen yogurt.

The important thing to remember is the necessity for variety and balance each day in foods selected from the Basic Four Food Groups. To complement a fast-food meal, the other meals should include adequate amounts of the vitamins, minerals, and fiber found in whole-grain breads and cereals, dark green leafy and yellow vegetables, legumes and fresh fruit.

Isn't it an unhealthy practice for school cafeterias to offer fast-food fare?

In order to increase food acceptance and decrease food waste, many school food service directors have capitalized on the popularity of fast foods among students. Reports show that the use of fast foods has increased participation in school lunch programs and decreased both food waste and cost per student. As long ago as 1973, for example, Len Fredrick, then the school food service director for Clark County, Nevada, incorporated fast foods into his luncheon menu. He succeeded in doubling school lunch participation at the secondary level, tripling the number of hot lunches bought by high school students, drastically reducing food waste, and lowering the price of the lunches.

Many fast foods contain ingredients that are high in both quality and nutritional value, and the total nutrient content of a fast-food lunch can contribute a significant proportion of nutrients to the overall diet. When included as part of a nutritionally balanced daily intake, fast foods can provide nutrients, energy, and fun. To quote Len Fredrick: "More good is derived from eating 100 percent of an almost nutritionally perfect meal than eating a little or none of a perfect meal."

Why deny yourself all of your fast-food favorites when, with the nutrition facts and a bit of common sense, you can enjoy them safely? After all, don't you deserve a break today?

Is it a good idea to ban all candy, soft drinks, and other sweets from the diets of children?

The key word in nutrition is *moderation*. Restricting choice does not teach moderation. Banning foods from the diets of children will not stop them from obtaining goodies else-where. Rather than promoting the ability to eat all foods moderately, attempts at restriction can lead to guilt associations with food, myths about "bad" foods, eating disorders, and food obsessions.

Parents can play a major role in the nutrition education of their children. Just as there are rules about bedtime hours and the use of radios and television sets, so should there be rules about what, when, and how much is eaten. Children should not be allowed to eat whatever they choose whenever they happen to think of it—and in unlimited amounts. Drinking apple juice and eating raisins all day long wouldn't do much for a child's nutritional status, dental health, or body weight, even though these are wise food selections to include as part of a balanced diet plan.

Eating is not merely a biological event. It is one of life's greatest pleasures. There is no need to back up every item we eat with an elaborate scientific, medical, or nutritional rationale. Both fruit juices and soft drinks are good sources of water, and both have about the same amount of sugar. It is perfectly all right to eat some things simply because we enjoy them—at any age!

As long as snacks do not fill up children so they are unable to eat their next meal, and as long as sweets are included as minor components of well balanced meals, there is no reason for healthy children to avoid enjoyable "junk foods." If children are overweight, foods rich in fats and sugars are the first foods to limit, but it is not necessary to prohibit them completely. Instead, overweight children should be encouraged to exercise more to help use up the extra calories they consume.

Don't Americans generally make poor food choices?

Many people who wonder about this seem to think that most Americans live on sweets, salty snack foods, and soft drinks. Perhaps this myth exists because these food items are constantly advertised on television. Actually, today's consumers funnel more of their food dollars into high-protein foods such as meat, poultry, fish, eggs, and dairy products. And these days, there is a wide array of more nutritious or lower-calorie versions of popular snack foods for nutrition-conscious shoppers to choose from. These include dry roasted nuts, salt-free chips, whole-grain crackers, sugar-free soft drinks, and desserts made with whole grains and dried fruit. Frozen-food choices include fruit-juice popsicles, sorbet, and low-fat frozen yogurt. There are even nutritious prepared dips, such as hummus (mashed chickpeas), guacamole (made from avocados), and babaganous (an eggplant variation).

It is quite interesting to see what people buy when they shop for food. Most people we have observed at a typical supermarket choose a variety of foods, including significant amounts of fruits, vegetables, enriched and whole grain breads and cereals, lean meats, poultry, fish, skim milk, low-fat cheeses, yogurt, and cottage cheese—as well as the various popular snack foods.

Not all foods are designed to provide only good nutrition. Some foods are meant for us to sit back and savor. Do you think that foods that provide energy, nutrients, taste, and fun should be considered "junky"? Remember that eating is more than just a physical necessity. It's all right to enjoy it.

7

The Truth About Food Additives

The Federal Food, Drug, and Cosmetic Act defines the term "food additive" as any substance that reasonably can be expected to become a component—or otherwise affect the characteristics—of any food. This means that any natural or synthetic substance added intentionally or accidentally to any food is considered a food additive.

The Food Protection Committee of the Food and Nutrition Board of the National Research Council defines a food additive as "a substance or mixture of substances, other than a basic foodstuff, which is present in food as a result of any aspect of production, processing, storage or packaging."

Some food additives are manufactured in laboratories, while others are derived from natural sources. The synthetic additives are often chemically identical to natural food constituents. Examples include vitamins and minerals. Food additives from natural sources include lecithin from egg yolks and soybeans, and carotene from yellow fruits and vegetables.

Like most things in life, food additives are not 100 percent risk-free. But consumers face far greater dangers from improper food preparation and overeating than from additives. Without food additives, the variety and quality of today's food supply would be greatly diminished, the quantity available would be far less, and prices would be much higher.

This chapter explains the functions and benefits as well as the controversies surrounding today's food additives.

95

I've heard that our foods are loaded with additives. Is this true?

Food additives constitute less than one percent of the total amount of food consumed. All additives are rigidly evaluated for safety—which is not the case for most of the "natural" foods we eat. Some individuals have sensitivities to some additives, just as certain people are sensitive to certain common foods, but most Americans can enjoy a safe, varied diet without being concerned about the additives in their food.

Concerns about the food supply are nothing new. From biblical times, people have complained about the food available to them. In the past, fears have been focused on the safety of milk, meat, fish, coffee, certain vegetables and fruits, and other items common to our weekly shopping lists.

Are you suggesting that fear of additives is part of a historical trend?

Yes. Today's "panic in the pantry" phenomenon is just the latest chapter in the age-old (and thick!) history of food scares. The prospect of contracting disease or facing death has always created enough fear to ensure that any widely publicized warning or word-of-mouth scare will be considered seriously by some portion of a population. Fear can interfere with people's ability to examine ideas in a rational manner.

If you become concerned about the safety of a particular food or food additive, seek information from a qualified professional in the nutrition field.

Couldn't Americans get along perfectly well without using any food additives?

We could get along, but not well. Without additives, our food supply would revert to the old state of bakery freshness: good today, stale tomorrow.

Additives are used to enhance the color and flavor of foods. Most consumers prefer foods to appear appetizingly familiar. Thus, colors are added to many foods to enhance their esthetic appeal. A wide variety of natural food flavors exists, but some are not available in large enough quantities to meet public demands. For example, there is not enough natural flavoring available in the world to flavor the ice cream consumed in this country in a single year. So synthetic flavors are required.

Additives also help to preserve food and enhance its nutritional value. Without preservatives, products made from wheat, rye, potatoes, and many other foods would quickly spoil and could cause serious health problems. Food enrichment and fortification with nutrient additives (vitamins and minerals) have helped to almost eliminate nutritional-deficiency diseases in the United States.

Considering the facts, it isn't very sensible to favor items labeled "no additives" or "no preservatives." In fact, unpreserved products tend to become stale, rancid, and sometimes even dangerous long before their "unnatural"—and less costly—counterparts.

Why do so many people think that food additives are "bad" and that "natural" foods are safe?

Many people have been misled by "health food" promoters into thinking that additives have not been sufficiently tested and are simply used for the convenience and economic advantage of the food industry. Actually, scientists understand more about food additives than they know about the chemistry of food itself! This is because food additives, especially the newer ones, have survived rigid testing procedures not applied to the ingredients in natural products. (And don't forget, food scientists who supervise food processing eat food too.) Additives that prove unsafe are legally banned from our food supply.

How are additives approved for use in our food supply?

Any substance newly proposed for addition to food must undergo strict testing. Details must be presented to the FDA about the chemical composition of the new additive, the manufacturing process, and the methods used to detect and measure its presence in food at the levels of expected use. Data must establish that the proposed testing methods are sufficiently sensitive to ensure compliance with appropriate regulations.

There also must be data to establish that the additive in question will accomplish the intended physical or technical effect in the food in which it is used and that the amount proposed for use is no higher than that required to accomplish this effect. Finally, the additive must be proven safe for its intended use. This requires scientific evidence from feeding studies and other tests using the proposed additive at various levels in the diet of two or more species of animals.

How is the "safe dose" of an additive determined?

"Sola dosis facit venenum"—"Only the dose makes the poison"—has been a basic principle of toxicology for centuries. Many substances used in small quantities as drugs are toxic in larger amounts. Arsenic, which was used to treat syphilis until penicillin was discovered, is one example. Curare, a deadly poison used by certain South American Indians, has been used in small amounts as a muscle relaxant; and the heart stimulant digitalis has saved thousands more lives than it ever threatened as part of the poisonous foxglove plant.

"Safe" is a relative term. Pre-clearance testing procedures ensure that the lowest effective level of an additive is used, and extensive animal tests—along with years of use by human volunteers—are required as evidence that this level is safe. Our food laws ensure that no substance found to pose even a slight risk to human or animal will be approved as an additive. The allowable percentage of the substance in the human diet is set at $1/100$ of the no-adverse-effect level in animals—a hundredfold margin of safety.

What is the "GRAS" list?

Certain substances which have been added to food for many years and are "Generally Recognized As Safe" by qualified scientists are exempt from the expensive premarketing clearance required for food additives. The GRAS list, published by the FDA, includes about seven hundred chemicals used before January 1, 1958, without any evidence of health hazard. Some familiar items are sugar, salt, vinegar and various common spices. The GRAS list was recently reevaluated.

If new data on a food chemical indicate a possible health risk, the FDA may revoke its GRAS classification of the substance and relabel it as an unapproved food additive. The agency can then require that a series of experiments be conducted to determine whether the chemical is safe for its intended use. If these tests support the suspicions, the FDA can prohibit or restrict use of the chemical.

Aren't there an awful lot of chemicals in today's foods?

There always have been and always will be chemicals in foods because all foods are composed of chemicals. Potatoes, for example, contain more than 150 distinct chemical substances. All "natural" foods are composed of complex chemicals, as are modern-day processed products. Of the 1,500 pounds of food eaten each year by the average consumer, 10 percent can be considered "additives," but most of this is herbs, spices, sugar, and salt. The other two-thousand-plus additives are consumed at a total annual rate of only ten pounds or so per person and include baking powder, yeast, carbon dioxide, and vitamin C, as well as artificial flavors and colors.

**Do food additives pose the greatest health
risks of all possible food hazards we face today?**

No! Contrary to popular opinion, FDA officials have ranked the food hazards faced by our society in the following order:

1. *Microbiological hazards.* Organisms that result in food poisoning affect some ten million people annually. Most cases are the result of improper handling of food in the kitchen, both at home and in restaurants. Several thousand Americans die from this hazard every year.

2. *Nutritional hazards.* These include overconsumption, poor food choices, poverty, indifference and ignorance.

3. *Environmental contaminants.* PCBs, mercury, and other heavy metals are about $^1/_{1000}$ as significant as the above factors in terms of known human effects. Human deaths from such contaminants have not bee reported.

4. *Natural toxicants in foods.* Nature's own poisons are a significant cause of human illness and death. Problem foods include certain mushrooms, herbs and fish.

5. *Pesticide residues and food additives.* Synthetic toxicants are estimated to be much less significant than the above-mentioned factors.

**Are all natural foods safe, or do some
contain potentially harmful chemicals?**

If all foods that contain traces of poisons, toxins, or cancer-causing agents were banned or severely restricted, we would all starve to death! Natural foods, like processed foods, are composed of chemicals. And most chemicals can pose health threats—depending, of course, on the dose ingested.

Would you like to eat something composed of the following ingredients: water, triglycerides of stearic, palmitic, oleic and linoleic acids, myosin, actin, glycogen, collagen, lecithin, cholesterol, urea, dipotassium phosphate, myoglobin, and many other chemicals?

No? What's the matter, don't you like steak?

Would you drink a beverage whose label listed the following components: acetone, methylacetate, furan, diacetyl, butanol, methylfuran, isoprene, methylbutanol, caffeine, dimethyl sulfide, essential oils, methanol, acetaldehyde, methylformate, ethanol, propionaldehyde, and many other chemicals?

No? Perhaps you don't drink coffee. The above is only a partial list of the hundreds of natural chemicals in this popular beverage and in many other foods.

Foods are composed of chemicals, and so is the human body. So, not all chemicals are "bad," whether natural or synthetic. In fact, many very poisonous chemicals are naturally present in our foods, while some of the chemicals most important for our health and safety are synthesized in the laboratory.

Richard Hall, Ph.D., former president of the Institute of Food Technologists, set forth the following menu to illustrate how consumption of natural toxins is inevitable:

Appetizer	*Food Contains*
Carrots	Carotatoxin (nerve poison)
	Myristicin (hallucinogen, also found in nutmeg)
Radishes	Two goitrogens (promote goiter by interference with iodine uptake)
Onions	Anti-thyroid chemicals
Olives	Tannins (cause cancer in animals)
	Benzo-(a)-pyrene (potent cancer-causing agent)
Main Course	
Shrimp	Arsenic (40–170 parts per million)
Potatoes	Solanine (interferes with nerve transmission)
Parsley	Myristicin (hallucinogen)
Wine	Alcohol (dehydrates, damages liver)
Dessert	
Cheese	Pressor amines (elevate blood pressure)
Bananas	Pressor amines (elevate blood pressure)
Tea	Tannins (damage intestinal lining)

The key to potential dangers from both natural foods and chemical additives is dose. If you ingest a large enough amount of almost any food, your body might be affected by any toxins naturally (or artificially) present. Obviously the best bet is "safety in numbers": eating a wide variety of foods in moderate amounts to ensure safe levels of intake of both undesired chemicals and desired nutrients.

This doesn't mean that we should avoid these menu items or other foods containing natural toxicants. You can safely enjoy moderate amounts of a varied menu of foods containing the vast array of food additives and naturally occurring chemical components. Your biggest concerns should be overeating and the accompanying hazards of overweight.

Does the FDA regulate the cancer-causing substances that are naturally present in our food?

Only a few. A double standard exists in our current chemical-evaluation procedures for foods. Aflatoxins, for example, are poisonous chemicals produced by certain molds that can grow on peanuts, rice, rye, corn, wheat, and other foods kept under certain conditions. The cancer-causing effects of these molds have been demonstrated in turkeys, rabbits, guinea pigs, dogs, cattle, ducks, fish, rhesus monkeys, and mice. In 1960, thousands of turkeys in England died of "turkey disease" caused by aflatoxin molds. Around the same time, in the northwestern United States, thousands of rainbow trout died from liver tumors believed to be caused by aflatoxins. In certain parts of Africa, where liver cancer is the most common male malignancy, aflatoxin-infested ground nuts (peanuts) are commonly used as a condiment. Therefore, the FDA and food manufacturers inspect peanut products for human and animal consumption and reject batches with unacceptably high contents of aflatoxin mold. Corn and corn products are deemed acceptable with aflatoxins up to 20 parts per billion. Thus, the amounts of aflatoxin in our food supply do not pose a significant health risk. The FDA tolerates some of this natural carcinogen but bans all "artificial" cancer-causing agents in foods.

It would be impossible to ban everything that conceivably could be unsafe. Instead, we must learn to live safely with known carcinogens by exposing ourselves to a low dose and accepting the fact that our environment cannot be 100 percent safe or free of carcinogens. Any chemical known or suspected to cause cancer, however, should be carefully monitored—and this includes "natural" aflatoxins as well as certain food additives. It is time for our society to enter a new age of reasonable methods for coping with the chemicals in our lives. Our current food chemical regulations should be revised and a consistent regulatory approach to both natural and synthetic chemicals should be adopted.

What is the Delaney Clause? Is it a practical way to protect us against food-induced cancers?

The Delaney Clause prohibits the use of any food additive in any amount found by appropriate tests to induce cancer in animals or humans. It was enacted in 1958 with the hope of reducing the potential cancer risks associated with food. It does not apply to naturally occurring toxins, additives sanctioned prior to 1958, unavoidable environmental contaminants, or GRAS food chemicals.

When the Clause was enacted, freeing our food supply from potential cancer hazards was thought to be a realistic goal. The only identified cancer risks at that time were those associated with certain man-made chemicals. However, as scientists developed the ability to detect smaller and smaller quantities of chemicals, they discovered that our food supply contains extremely small amounts of many carcinogens and other toxins, both natural and synthetic. In light of this knowledge, we and many others believe that the Delaney Clause is too rigid. The National Academy of Sciences and the American Council on Science and Health have recommended that it be modified to make our food safety policy more appropriate and practical.

How much risk is involved in consuming saccharin?

In 1977, the FDA announced its intention to ban saccharin as a food additive in diet foods and beverages. The agency based its decision on the results of a single study in which high doses of saccharin caused bladder tumors in rats. The proposed action was so vigorously challenged by scientists and consumers that Congress blocked further regulatory action. Saccharin-containing products are required to carry a warning label:

USE OF THIS PRODUCT MAY BE HAZARDOUS TO YOUR HEALTH. THIS PRODUCT CONTAINS SACCHARIN WHICH HAS BEEN DETERMINED TO CAUSE CANCER IN LABORATORY ANIMALS.

Unless the Congressional moratorium ends, consumers can weigh for themselves the benefits and risks of consuming saccharin.

What evidence is there that saccharin is unsafe? Have any human studies confirmed that saccharin causes cancer?

Since 1950, more than twenty long-term experiments with saccharin have been conducted using rats, mice, hamsters, and monkeys. At least seventeen provided either negative or inconclusive evidence of any possible cancer-causing potential. In the three other tests, a small number of the male rats exposed to the largest doses of saccharin—from the time they were conceived through adulthood—developed bladder tumors. We doubt, however, that these results indicate a need for further research in this area.

More than a dozen studies with saccharin have been conducted on humans, but only one indicated any possible risk. Most experts have severely criticized the design of this study, and three larger studies failed to confirm any such risk. Remember that carcinogens are all around us; occasional exposure to small doses does not cause cancer, but consistent exposure to large doses that exceed individual tolerance levels may result in cancer. Dosage and tolerance are the main factors to consider in determining cancer risk for both animals and humans.

What do most nutritionists advise regarding saccharin use?

The prevailing opinion is that there is no proof of health hazard to consumers at current levels of use. The availability of other artificial sweeteners (aspartame and acesulfame-K) has reduced any public dependence on saccharin while permitting its continued use in the products for which it is best suited.

What is your opinion of aspartame?

Aspartame, a chemical compound composed mainly of two amino acids (phenylalanine and aspartic acid), is approved by the FDA for use in beverages and several other foodstuffs. Individuals with phenylketonuria (PKU), a rare metabolic disorder, must avoid products containing phenylalanine. Some individuals have reported headaches, dizziness, stomach upsets, and various other symptoms after exposure to aspartame. But double-blind tests suggest the symptoms are either coincidental or placebo effects. In the amounts generally consumed, aspartame is a safe alternative to sugar-sweetened products.

Are saccharin or aspartame helpful in weight reduction?

No long-term study indicates that either is helpful. Large-scale studies using sugar substitutes have failed to demonstrate any weight-loss benefit associated with either saccharin or aspartame. One study examining the weight changes of over 78,000 women found that those who used artificial sweeteners were more likely to *gain* weight. Users of these products tend to make up for the deleted sugar-calories by consuming additional foodstuffs. Some researchers believe that artificial sweeteners trigger sugar cravings and stimulate the appetite, actually causing consumers to eat more.

Is the nitrite in bacon and other processed foods dangerous?

Nitrites have been used as food additives for hundreds of years without any detectable ill effects in humans. The amounts used in bacon and other cured meats (less than 5 percent of our total nitrite intake) are so small that they are considered insignificant by most scientists. The main dietary source of nitrite is actually the nitrate present in many vegetables. Nitrate is rapidly changed to nitrite by the bacteria normally present in the mouth. Nitrate is naturally abundant in spinach, beets, radishes, eggplant, celery, lettuce, collards, turnip greens, and about half of U.S. water sources.

About 80 percent of the nitrite in the body is found in the saliva. Nitrites react with amines present in the stomach and intestine to form nitrosamines. It is nitrosamines, rather than nitrates or nitrites, that are carcinogenic in animals, but only in high concentrations. The amounts of nitrosamines that form in humans who eat bacon or other nitrite- or nitrate-containing foods is minimal. Thus, bacon is not a harmful food for that reason—but be aware of its high saturated fat content.

Why are nitrites added to certain foods?

Nitrite is added to bacon, ham, hot dogs, other cured meats, and some fish because it provides the pleasant taste and familiar colors we associate with such products. However, its main function is as a preservative—to prevent the development of the deadly botulism toxin. So far, the FDA has not banned the use of nitrites, because the benefits outweigh any possible risks. However, the meat industry did voluntarily reduce the amount of nitrite used in processed products and added ascorbic acid (vitamin C), which greatly reduces the formation of nitrosamines.

Do food additives, such as artificial colorings and flavorings, make children fidgety?

In 1973, Benjamin Feingold, M.D., chief of the allergy department of the Kaiser-Permanente Medical Center in Oakland, California, issued a book called *Why Your Child Is Hyperactive.* He claimed that the major cause in children is food additives, mainly artificial flavorings and colorings, plus the chemical salicylate. Salicylates are found in many medications and foods, including aspirin, apples, apricots, cherries, grapes, nectarines, oranges, peaches, plums, prunes, raisins, raspberries, strawberries, tomatoes, and cucumbers.

The Feingold diet eliminates virtually all processed foods, such as soft drinks, ice cream, candy, baked goods, processed cheese, luncheon meats, hot dogs, margarine—even toothpaste. Most condiments must be avoided, and convenience foods are restricted. Dining in school cafeterias, restaurants, fast food outlets, and even in other people's homes can be difficult for children on the diet. Homemade foods prepared from "scratch" become a requirement for all family meals. Dr. Feingold advised that his diet be followed by all family members so that the hyperactive child will not feel "different." This is a lot of work for a homemaker, and quite a project for any family to take on.

The diet itself probably has little if any effect. All of the large-scale studies have failed to prove that salicylates or artificial colors and flavors have the dramatic impact on hyperactivity that Dr. Feingold claimed. If these chemicals do affect behavior, the relationship is minor. Only a few hyperactive children, perhaps a fraction of one percent, may experience a mildly adverse reaction to one or several artificial colors or flavors present in foods. There is no reason for school food services or food manufacturers to change their methods in an effort to prevent or control hyperactivity.

If diet is not the cause of hyperactive behavior, why do many parents believe that the Feingold diet has helped their children?

Hyperactivity (also called "hyperkinesis" or "attention deficit disorder") is characterized by a variety of symptoms. Hyperactive children may be restless, excitable, easily distracted, and/or emotionally unstable, as well as irritable, aggressive, disruptive, and uncoordinated. Many school-age children in America have been labeled "hyperactive," but this label is too loosely applied.

Conventional treatment for hyperactive children includes counseling and/or medication. The Feingold theory is attractive to parents because it offers a "natural" alternative to drug therapy and allows them to shift the "blame" for their children's behavior from faulty parenting to processed food.

Research scientists who have analyzed the use of diet therapy in hyperactivity have discovered what most parents fail to recognize: adherence to the diet regimen causes significant changes in family relationships and lifestyle that can affect the child's behavior. The increased attention alone can result in a reduction in hyperactivity. In addition, the child's own sense of self-responsibility may grow as a result of taking charge of food choices at school, friends' homes, and social events—and this may help to quell immature behavior. Still, any possible benefits should be weighed against the potential harm of instilling in children the false belief that their behavior is controlled primarily by what they eat.

What are BHA and BHT? Are they dangerous?

BHA and BHT are the abbreviations for butylated hydroxyanisole and butylated hydroxytoluene, two antioxidants added to many foods including margarine, snack foods, crackers, and breakfast cereals. These additives are safe in the concentrations used in processed foods. They are used to prevent "off" flavors, retain crispness, and preserve nutrient content.

Some research indicates that BHA and BHT may actually play an important role in the prevention of stomach cancer. When they are added to the diet of laboratory animals, there is a marked reduction in stomach cancer. Some cancer epidemiologists believe that part of the decline in the human death rate from this type of cancer since the 1940s—when the widespread use of BHA and BHT began—may be a result of increased use of these two additives. Despite this, their use has been reduced by pressure from certain consumer activists.

I understand that food irradiation is regulated by the FDA as a "food additive." Does it pose any dangers?

Beginning in the the 1950s, irradiation has been used in some thirty-five countries to help preserve foods. We believe it is safe and potentially very valuable to our society. The process uses ionizing radiation (electrically charged particles) to kill organisms that might spoil foods, thereby prolonging the useful life of these foods. Irradiation does *not* make foods radioactive. In 1981 the World Health Organization concluded that "all the toxicological studies carried out on a large number of irradiated foods . . . have produced no evidence of adverse effects." Although the FDA has approved the use of irradiation of fresh fruits, vegetables, pork, poultry, dried herbs, and spices, vocal opposition by consumer groups has made manufacturers reluctant to market irradiated products. So far its use in the United States has been limited to commercial spices and seasonings. However, a company in Florida is now building a facility for irradiating fruits, vegetables, and poultry.

What is MSG? Does it cause "Chinese Restaurant Syndrome"?

MSG is the abbreviation for monosodium glutamate, a flavor-enhancer used for over two thousand years. MSG is the sodium salt of glutamic acid, an amino acid abundant in both plant and animal protein, including the protein of the human body). The average amount of glutamic consumed daily is about $1/1000$ of the amount found in the human body, and most of it comes from natural foods rather than added MSG.

MSG was first isolated from seaweed in Japan and is now produced from sugar beets and by the fermentation of molasses. It is a fine, white, crystalline product similar in appearance to table salt but containing only 12 percent sodium—about one third the amount in table salt. Because research suggests that sodium may play a role in the development of high blood pressure in predisposed individuals, MSG may be useful as a salt substitute.

Hundreds of studies conducted on humans and laboratory animals furnish reliable evidence that MSG is safe for most people when consumed in moderate amounts. It does appear to cause unpleasant effects in sensitive individuals, especially when it is absorbed rapidly—as may occur at the beginning of a meal when the stomach is empty. This is most likely to happen when one consumes a broth-type soup as the first course (often the case with a Chinese meal). In susceptible individuals, the following symptoms may appear: dizziness, headache, chest pain, heart palpitation, weakness, nausea, vomiting, a burning sensation, and a feeling of tightness and/or numbness in the upper chest, neck, or face. Symptoms can persist for several hours. MSG sensitivity is commonly referred to as the "Chinese Restaurant Syndrome." Individuals who believe they are sensitive to MSG can check food labels to avoid foods that contain this additive. Most restaurants will refrain from using it if requested to do so.

What about sulfites?

Sulfites have been used in many foods and wines to slow spoilage. Until a few years ago, they were widely used in restaurant salad bars to prevent the browning of fresh fruits and vegetables, potatoes, dips such as guacamole, and other popular restaurant fare. Unfortunately, it was discovered that sulfites can cause allergic reactions that are severe or even fatal, particularly in people with asthma. The FDA has taken steps to restrict their use and is reviewing whether they should remain classified as GRAS. The National Restaurant Association has asked its members to discontinue using sulfites. Most restaurants have complied. Sulfites pose a real danger only to some individuals who are asthmatic or who tend to be highly allergic. It is noteworthy that sulfites are the only additives that have proven dangerous among several thousand that have been used in recent years.

If additives aren't "poisonous chemicals," does this mean that pesticides are equally safe?

Pesticides are poisonous chemicals, and that's why they are effective. They are poisonous for weeds, insects, worms, rats, and other pests. But strictly enforced regulations and tolerance levels minimize the hazard to humans from ingesting the pesticide residues normally found on foods.

Some so-called "health foods" and "organically grown" produce actually contain as much or more pesticide residue than do regular supermarket products. So there is no reason to pay inflated prices due to fears about pesticides. Pesticides are unsafe only if they are handled carelessly or consumed in large quantities. The amounts in the American diet are extremely small and are not harmful.

So contemporary Americans should not be worried about additives and pesticides?

That's correct. The fear that foods may cause diseases has always existed. The media have elevated this fear with scare stories about our food supply. A few years ago the *New England Journal of Medicine* published an enlightening editorial entitled "Cancer! Alarm! Cancer!" which stated: "American cancerophobia, in brief, is a disease as serious to society as cancer is to the individual—and morally more devastating." The editorial concluded that, just as no one has the right to shout "fire" in a crowded theater, no one should have the right to stand up in our cancerophobic society and cry "Cancer!" without adequate cause. Nor should anyone publicly deride any food additive or foodstuff without adequate evidence to back up the criticism.

The current fear of "chemicals" is a double-barreled source of concern. First, the antichemical approach overlooks the taste, safety, and esthetic benefits offered by food additives. Second, preoccupation with unknown side effects of food chemicals may distract consumers from the known health threats of cigarette smoking, lack of exercise, overeating, and excessive stress.

So let's step ahead and work towards good health and total fitness by eating a well-balanced diet, maintaining a reasonable body weight, exercising regularly, and avoiding unnecessary stress—including needless fears about food additives, pesticides, and other chemicals in our foods. Why not relax and enjoy the many different safe, nutritious, and delicious foods that our modern marketplace makes available?

8

Practical Weight Control

Thin has not always been "in." Look at Venus de Milo, Cleopatra, Marilyn Monroe, and the "full-figured" Jane Russell. The stout male build also was once admired, the excess flab regarded a sign of wealth and leisure. Historically, body fat symbolized fertility, prosperity, and "the good life"—free from common concerns about not having enough to eat. Today, however, more than a quarter of America's adults are considered overweight, and getting rid of excess body fat has become a national obsession. A multibillion dollar diet industry is thriving. Crash diets are featured in most women's magazines. Books touting quick weight-loss schemes are found on bestseller lists. Weight-loss clinics and inches-off salons are cropping up everywhere. And sales of diet pills, diet foods, diet drinks, and other gimmicks are booming.

Waist-watchers, beware! Ignore hollow dietary promises and irrational weight-loss claims. If you need to lose weight, choose a sensible diet-and-exercise program you can follow for life—a longer, healthier, happier life.

Are obesity and overweight the same thing?

Strictly speaking, obesity refers to an excess accumulation of fatty tissue in the body, while overweight refers to weight greater than that

110

listed in an established height-weight table. Overweight is commonly defined as from 10 to 20 percent above the weights in the Metropolitan Life Insurance Company tables (see below), while obesity has been defined as 20 percent or more above these weights. Since most overweight people are overfat, the terms "obesity" and "overweight" are often used interchangeably.

What are the hazards of excess body weight?

Even though most dieters try to shed pounds for aesthetic reasons, there are definite health risks associated with being obese. The human body was not built to tote around a heavy overload, and it tends to wear out sooner when forced to do this. The following problems are associated with or aggravated by obesity:

heart attacks	strokes
high blood pressure	blood clots in the legs
varicose veins	hemorrhoids
diabetes	arthritis
kidney disorders	gout
gallstones	menstrual irregularities
reduced fertility	irritated skin patches
increased surgical risks	rashes
poor wound healing	decreased immunity
shorter lifespan	stretch marks
cancer of the breast, colon, uterus, and prostate	difficulties during pregnancy

How can I determine the best weight for me?

One way is to compare your present weight to the ranges provided in the desirable-weight tables. The term "desirable weight" was coined nearly half a century ago by Louis Dublin, a statistician at the Metropolitan Life Insurance Company. After grouping individuals by age, height, and weight, he found that those who lived the longest were the ones who maintained their weight at the average level for 25-year-olds. Since Dublin felt that there is no "ideal" weight for all individuals, he called these ranges "desirable weights."

Some statisticians have criticized these figures because they were obtained from a select sample of people: relatively healthy adults who qualified for life insurance. But they still appear to be sound data that relate weight to life expectancy. These tables were revised in 1983, increasing the weight ranges by a few pounds. Many health professionals, though, believe that the older weights (given in Table 8:1) are still the best ones to use. Muscular males, such as trained

Table 8:1. Desirable Weights for Men and Women of Age 25 and Over

Source: Metropolitan Life Insurance Company. Data are based on weights associated with lowest death rates. To obtain weight for adults younger than 25, subtract one pound for each year under 25.

	Height in Shoes	Small Frame	Medium Frame	Large Frame
Men	5'–2"	112–120	118–129	126–141
	5'–3"	115–123	121–133	129–144
	5'–4"	118–126	124–136	132–148
	5'–5"	121–129	127–139	135–152
	5'–6"	124–133	130–143	138–156
	5'–7"	128–137	134–147	142–161
	5'–8"	132–141	138–152	147–166
	5'–9"	136–145	142–156	151–170
	5'–10"	140–150	146–160	155–174
	5'–11"	144–154	150–165	159–179
	6'–0"	148–158	154–170	164–184
	6'–1"	152–162	158–175	168–189
	6'–2"	156–167	162–180	173–194
	6'–3"	160–171	167–185	178–199
	6'–4"	164–175	172–190	182–204
Women	4'–10"	92–98	96–107	104–119
	4'–11"	94–101	98–110	106–122
	5'–0"	96–104	101–113	109–125
	5'–1"	99–107	104–116	112–128
	5'–2"	102–110	107–119	115–131
	5'–3"	105–113	110–122	118–134
	5'–4"	108–116	113–126	121–138
	5'–5"	111–119	116–130	125–142
	5'–6"	114–123	120–135	129–146
	5'–7"	118–127	124–139	133–150
	5'–8"	122–131	128–143	137–154
	5'–9"	126–135	132–147	141–158
	5'–10"	130–140	136–151	145–163
	5'–11"	134–144	140–155	149–168
	6'–0"	138–148	144–159	153–173

Weight in Pounds (in Indoor Clothing)

athletes, may be *overweight* according to the tables without being overfat. Since muscle weighs a little more than fat, an active football player or a logger may weigh more than his sedentary peers, yet not require weight (fat) loss. Conversely, a sedentary person might not weigh above the desirable range, yet could be carrying too much body fat. Thus, weight tables provide only a rough guide and may not indicate whether a person is too fat.

If you need to lose weight, the following formulas can give you an approximate goal:

• *Women:* 100 pounds for the first 5 feet in height, plus 5 pounds for each additional inch.

• *Men:* 106 pounds for the first 5 feet, plus 6 pounds for each additional inch.

Is body fat of any benefit to modern-day humans?

Fat is stored fuel, once needed in large amounts to supply energy during times of famine. Primitive humans could not raid a refrigerator or drive to a 24-hour fast-food outlet whenever hunger pangs struck. When food was plentiful, our ancestors consumed large quantities so that their fat stores could provide energy when food was scarce. Modern-day humans who have access to ample amounts of food don't need to store large amounts of body fat in order to survive.

In proper amounts, however, fat is still important. Body fat provides insulation against the cold, protective padding for vital organs, and energy reserves for women to use as needed during pregnancy and breast-feeding. Fat—in moderate amounts—also gives the body contours that are aesthetically pleasing.

How do calories relate to body weight?

A calorie is a measurement of energy, used to describe the energy value of foods and the energy requirements of physical activity. For weight to be maintained, the amount of calories taken in as food must equal the amount of calories expended by the body in metabolic processes and physical activity. If you eat and drink more calories than you "burn," you will gain weight. If you "burn" more calories than you consume, you will lose weight.

A pound of body fat represents the storage of about 3,500 calories. To lose a pound, you need to create a 3,500-calorie deficit by taking in fewer calories and/or expending more. To shed this pound in a week's time, you could consume 500 fewer calories per day or burn off 500 more calories per day by exercising. The most effective method for weight loss is to combine the two approaches by consuming fewer calories and expending more through increased exercise.

What foods constitute a dieter's worst enemies?

A gram of dietary fat provides about 9 calories, whereas a gram of protein or carbohydrate yields only 4 calories. Alcohol offers about 7 calories per gram. (These figures per ounce would be 270, 120, and 210.) Vitamins, minerals, fiber, and water provide no calories. Thus, cutting back on high-fat foods and alcoholic beverages will enhance the weight-loss process.

The "dieter's worst enemies" are not specific foods, but the psychological strains that can accompany a restrictive diet. All foods can be included in a weight control program if consumed in moderation as part of a varied, well balanced diet with a total caloric intake low enough and a caloric output high enough to produce the desired weight loss. In fact, dieters are more apt to stick with a plan that allows freedom to enjoy the foods they like.

What diet plan do you advocate?

To be successful, a diet must be integrated into your lifestyle so that proper eating habits become permanent. The most sensible program is a well balanced low-fat diet—based on moderate servings of a variety of foods chosen from among and within the Basic Four Food Groups, and coupled with regular physical activity. Sound weight control is based on simple scientific facts—but this certainly does not mean that adopting such a program for a lifetime is an easy task. The sad statistics show that most weight-loss attempts end in failure, largely due to bouncing from one fad diet to another while searching for a magical cure for overweight.

If you are ready and willing to accept the facts, you can lose weight safely and effectively—and keep it off. First, check with your physician to make sure that you do not have any underlying health problem that would preclude a diet-and-exercise program at this time. Next, determine your desirable weight range and calculate the number of pounds you need to shed in order to reach it. Then draw up a reasonable time plan. Remember that it takes a 3,500-calorie deficit to lose one pound of body fat, so a daily deficit of 500 calories (accomplished by eating less and/or exercising more) will mean a weekly loss of one pound. Since exercise is a must, be sure your plan includes physical activities that you enjoy. Remember, too, that "crash dieting" doesn't work.

You may want to obtain counseling from a registered dietitian who specializes in weight control who can help you design a well-balanced, low-fat, low-alcohol plan that suits your lifestyle and personal needs. Or, if you prefer company while dieting, you may want to join a diet group. Weight Watchers and TOPS, for example, are reputable national programs that conduct local meetings in many communities. These organizations provide sane diet advice and strong peer support. Other programs should be carefully evaluated to ensure that their dietary advice is sensible and their staff is qualified. Be wary of highly advertised diet "clinics" that offer high-priced crash diets, particularly those that advocate liquid meal substitutes or other "special" foods.

If you decide to diet on your own, we suggest that you purchase a handbook on weight control from the reading list in Appendix C. Avoid the flashy fad diet books that promise an easy way out. If a diet plan sounds too good to be true, you can bet that it is! Be sure your diet plan includes a wide variety of foodstuffs, including a moderate amount of your own personal favorites. Very-low-calorie diets are nutritionally deficient, medically unsound, psychologically depressing, ultimately self-defeating, and sometimes even life-threatening. Dietary deprivation is harmful, both physically and emotionally.

Can you suggest how to modify behavior to enhance weight control?

The following tips may help you:

1. Use alternatives to food as rewards (for example, long walks, relaxing baths, tickets to a movie or play).

2. Serve yourself moderate portions of low-fat foods. Resist the temptation to always "clean the plate." Eat when you are hungry and stop eating when you are satisfied.

3. Whenever you are eating, ask yourself why. Is it because you are hungry or due to an "outside" cause? For example, do you eat in response to places or events from your past, so that vacationing near the ocean results in fried-clam binges every summer, or a winter cold

inevitably leads to mothering yourself with "comfort" foods?

4. Try not to eat simply as a response to the sight or smell of food, such as binging after a trip to the supermarket, gobbling fresh baked goods upon catching a whiff of the local bakery, or snacking in response to tempting TV or magazine ads.

5. Avoid fantasizing about foods. If you allow yourself to eat *moderate* portions of your favorites, you will be less apt to crave these foods and overindulge on them.

6. Avoid eating according to the clock. You do not have to have a doughnut just because it is coffee break time; noon does not automatically signal lunchtime; and midnight does not have to mean snack time.

7. Avoid eating while engaged in other activities. It is difficult to obtain the psychological satisfaction provided by food if you are absorbed in a television show, the newspaper, or in home or office work.

8. Select alternative outlets for emotions. Eat when you are physically hungry, but avoid food when you are emotionally "hungry" (bored, frustrated, anxious, stressed, lonely, etc.).

9. Avoid eating for the purpose of procrastination. Food should not be used as a diversion, a means for avoiding confrontations or escaping from duties.

10. Find places other than the kitchen where you can seek refuge from people who stir up your emotional "hunger." The next time your employer is driving you to drink, your children are driving you to the cookie jar, or your spouse is driving you to a fast-food binge, take a brisk walk or drop in on a friend. Just be sure to head away from the aggravating individual and the tempting foodstuffs!

How can I evaluate the various weight-loss programs available in my area?

A registered dietitian or your personal physician can help you determine what is most appropriate for you. A sound program will include a balanced diet, an exercise plan, behavior modification techniques for both weight loss and lifetime maintenance, all at a reasonable price. Don't just look at programs that are widely advertised. See what is offered by your local hospital dietary department, dietitians in private practice, and the longstanding conventional programs like Weight Watchers, Diet Workshop, and TOPS.

What can college students do to avoid the weight gain so common during the first year away from home?

Three things may help:
1. Plan menus in advance. By knowing ahead of time what you are going to eat, you can avoid making impulsive high-calorie, high-fat choices. Many college food services provide nutrition and caloric information to interested students, and some offer special diet menus.
2. Avoid overstocked dorm refrigerators. Confine meals and snacks to the dining hall, so you can avoid late-night refrigerator raids and frequent snacking during study times.
3. Try not to use eating as an excuse to procrastinate, a way to fill unoccupied time, or a basis for socializing. The stress-reducing and social aspects of food make it easy to substitute eating for studying, exercise, classes, conversation, even dates and friendship. Study-time "munchies" and tempting party fare can also lead to unwanted weight gain.

Thus, the best advice for fat-fearing college students is to avoid becoming too focused on food. If you and your dorm mates want low-fat milk or a salad bar in your dining hall, let the food service personnel know your wishes. At many colleges, a staff dietitian can help students with special dietary concerns, including weight reduction, vegetarianism, or other conditions requiring dietary modification.

Would it help to switch to "light" versions of favorite foods?

The "light" explosion in the marketplace has touched everything from beer and chips to cupcakes and pastries. Low-calorie soft drinks and low-fat milk products have assumed a significant place in the diet food market; now "light" foods are clamoring for a share. Yet there is no uniform definition of "light." Products so labeled may be reduced only in portion size or weight—or may have some other nutritionally insignificant characteristic. (For example, Sara Lee's original "Light Classic Desserts" were light in texture but had *more* calories than the traditional products.) If you wish to consider using "light" products, analyze their labels carefully to see whether they actually provide the caloric discounts you desire.

Can substituting fructose for table sugar help cut calories?

Before purchasing fructose sweeteners, it would be wise to weigh the supposed advantages against the costs. Fructose is used mostly in "dietetic" foods, especially those intended for diabetics, while crystalline fructose and high-fructose corn syrup are increasingly used in processed foods and beverages. There is no evidence to support the use of fructose as a weight-reducing aid. Fructose provides the same number of calories per serving as sucrose (table sugar). Since it is somewhat sweeter than sucrose, lesser amounts of fructose might be needed to sweeten certain foods. However, when fructose is added to hot drinks, baked in foods, or mixed with non-acidic products, some of the sweetening power is lost. Fructose is discussed further in Chapter 10.

Is fasting an effective way to lose weight?

Fasting produces rapid weight loss, but most of the initial loss is body water—which is regained as soon as normal eating is resumed. In addition to being dangerous, fasting does nothing to help people change their undesirable eating habits so that they can achieve and maintain a desirable weight. In fact, many individuals who fast will binge when they resume eating, because the temporary deprivation has exaggerated their appetite. Researchers have found that self-induced starvation stimulates a physical as well as psychological drive to eat—and overeat.

Does dieting shrink the stomach?

Contrary to popular myth, dieting does not shrink the stomach. The average stomach holds 1½ to 2 quarts of food and beverage. It can expand a bit in order to hold this amount or a little more, but it will not remain permanently extended due to overeating. Nor will it shrivel up from undereating. The inclusion of bulky, fiber-containing foods (fruits, vegetables, whole grain breads, and cereals) is desirable during weight-loss attempts—or at any other time—because they are filling yet low in fat. On the other hand, many fad diets cause bloating and other gastrointestinal distress.

Did anyone ever starve to death from dieting?

Aside from the casualties resulting from "anorexia nervosa" (discussed in Chapter 12), relatively few deaths have been attributed solely to dieting. One of the most widely publicized of the potentially deadly diet plans was the appropriately-named "Last Chance Diet." This liquid protein regime was popularized in the late 1970s in a book by osteopath Dr. Robert Linn. Dieters were restricted to about 400 calories per day from a low-quality protein powder made from beef hides and cow underbellies. The FDA documented over fifty deaths associated with the use of liquid protein diets, including some in which the protein was of high quality. Some of these deaths—in healthy individuals—resulted from sudden heart stoppage secondary to metabolic imbalance. The moral of this story is that unbalanced, extreme diets can be dangerous, even fatal.

What about today's very-low-calorie (VLC) diets?

VLC diets ("protein-sparing modified fasts") typically contain 600 to 800 calories per day, most of them from high-quality proteins, plus vitamins and minerals, particularly potassium. Some programs use liquid formulas, while others utilize food sources (poultry, fish, and lean meats).

Total fasting throws the body into a state of ketosis, in which the body burns not only its fat stores but protein from lean body mass—muscles and major organs such as the heart and kidneys. Prolonged fasting can also lead to anemia, impairment of liver function, kidney stones, mineral imbalances, and other adverse effects. For this reason, properly designed VLC diets include enough protein and other nutrients to prevent the body from cannibalizing its own lean tissue.

Because of their potential danger, programs this drastic should be restricted to individuals who are at least 30 percent overweight and should include a weekly examination by a physician, blood tests to detect potentially dangerous metabolic abnormalities, and behavior modification. In controlled experiments, patients have typically consumed the diets for twelve to sixteen weeks. Weight gain is common after the eating of food is resumed, but it is more likely to occur with do-it-yourself programs than with medically supervised ones.

Can any prescription drug help curb my appetite?

Amphetamines ("speed") were once widely prescribed as an appetite suppressant. Their adverse effects far outweigh any usefulness as a diet aid, but a few physicians—contrary to prevailing medical opinion—still prescribe them. Amphetamines are physically and psychologically addicting. Although they can temporarily suppress appetite, tolerance develops and increasingly higher dosages must be used.

The body's thyroid hormones help to control metabolism—the rate at which calories are used up by the body. Unless the body's supply is deficient, addition of small amounts of thyroid supplements will suppress normal thyroid hormone production and thus have no lasting metabolic effect. Large dosages can cause weight reduction, but they can also raise blood pressure and strain the heart. Doctors who prescribe high dosages of thyroid hormone in the absence of thyroid deficiency should be investigated by state licensing authorities to determine whether they should be permitted to remain in practice.

Human chorionic gonadotropin (HCG) is a hormone found in the urine of pregnant women. HCG has been claimed to mobilize stored fat and suppress appetite, but there is no scientific evidence to support these claims. A few "clinics" administer weekly injections of HCG and put their clients on a very-low-calorie diet. The diet, of course, will cause temporary weight loss but may also result in loss of protein from vital organs.

Fenfluramine has been shown to be an effective appetite suppressant. Unfortunately, once the drug is stopped, the lost weight rapidly reappears. Fenfluramine's adverse effects include diarrhea, drowsiness, high blood pressure, and glaucoma. Thus, unless one is willing to undergo Fenfluramine therapy indefinitely—under careful medical supervision—and risk the potential dangers, this diet drug is also a poor choice.

Mazindol is also prescribed as an appetite suppressant. Although it is not an amphetamine derivative, it does stimulate the nervous system. Its appetite-quelling effects tend to diminish with time, so that it gradually becomes ineffective as a weight-loss aid.

As yet, there is no prescription drug that can effectively curb appetite without causing undesirable side effects. Moreover, none can help to permanently alter the poor eating habits that cause overweight. Only you can do that.

What about nonprescription "diet aids"?

Many advertised diet pills contain phenylpropanolamine (PPA), a nasal decongestant included in some cold remedies. Although PPA will cause appetite to diminish temporarily if administered in large amounts, it appears to be ineffective as an appetite suppressant when taken in small (safe) dosages. The adverse effects of PPA include headaches, blurred vision, sweating, rapid pulse, nervousness, insomnia, dizziness, heart palpitations, and elevations in blood pressure. PPA should never be used by pregnant and nursing women, young children or the elderly, or by anyone with high blood pressure, heart disease, diabetes, or thyroid or kidney disorders.

Other supposed "diet pills" contain caffeine, for "pep," and/or benzocaine to numb the taste buds. Some contain bulk-forming ingredients that supposedly expand in the stomach to cause a "full" feeling. Certain "diet aids" are little more than candy-like vitamin/mineral supplements. Eating these candies shortly before meals is claimed to "spoil the appetite," but this seldom happens.

Mail-order diet pills are typically advertised with claims like, "Melts fat away . . . 2 pounds gone the first 24 hours . . . 10 pounds gone the first 7 days!" Unfortunately for desperate dieters, none of these products is effective as a weight-reduction aid. They may be sold with a low-calorie diet plan that can bring about weight reduction, but most of these diets are not nutritionally balanced.

What about weight-loss products sold through "health food" stores?

One such product sold in tablet form is glucomannan, a dietary fiber extracted from konjac, a Japanese root plant. This substance is a bulk-forming agent. When consumed prior to meals, glucomannan will expand in the stomach to provide a feeling of "fullness." Unfortunately, most overweight individuals do not always stop eating when they feel full. If they did, they would probably not be overweight. Double-blind testing has demonstrated no benefit from including glucomannan in a weight-control program. Glucomannan products have also been promoted for lowering cholesterol, eliminating ingested chemicals, aiding digestion, and reducing blood sugar levels. However, there is no scientific evidence to support these claims.

Pectin has been marketed in powder and tablet form as a "wonder drug" for desperate weight watchers. These products do not promote weight loss but can cause flatulence and diarrhea. Pectin is a form of fiber found naturally in apples, apricots, plums, the rinds of citrus fruits, and root vegetables such as carrots and radishes. Including such foods in your diet can provide beneficial amounts of fiber with minimal risk of adverse effects.

Spirulina maxima is a blue-green alga, a dietary staple in some parts of the world. Spirulina contains protein of poor quality plus certain other nutrients, all of which can be obtained much less expensively from conventional foods. Despite claims for weight-loss benefits, spirulina has no value as a diet aid.

"Starch blockers" were once common on the shelves of "health food" stores. Made from enzymes extracted from beans, these products were claimed to be able to prevent digestion of significant amounts of dietary starch when taken before mealtime. Yet the body produces more starch-digesting enzymes than these pills could possibly block. And since enzymes are proteins, they are digested soon after being taken by mouth. Moreover, when undigested starch reaches the large intestine, it is fermented by bacteria normally present, producing gas and intestinal cramps. Some users of starch blockers were reported to have abdominal pain, nausea, vomiting, and diarrhea. After concluding that "starch blockers" were unsafe, the FDA ordered them off the market and secured court orders against companies that defied the order.

Unfortunately, the market for "magic" diet pills and the imaginations of those who concoct them are virtually unlimited. After "starch blockers" disappeared, several companies began advertising products falsely claimed to block fat, calories, or sugar from being absorbed. Perhaps the most notorious was *Cal-Ban 3000,* a guar gum product that swells by absorbing water. After cases were reported in which the product caused complete blockage of the esophagus—forcing users to seek emergency hospital care—state and federal agencies stopped its sales.

**I've seen ads for pills that are claimed
to cause weight loss while you sleep.
What's in them? Do they work?**

These pills contain amino acids that are claimed to cause weight loss by releasing growth hormone. These claims are based on misinterpretations of experiments in which animals given injections of large amounts were observed to eat less food. Government enforcement actions have driven many "growth-hormone releasers" from the marketplace, but a few remain.

Can any special psychological techniques help reduce the urge to eat?

Hypnotists guide their clients into a trancelike state and then offer them subconscious suggestions, such as "You will never eat chocolate cake again" or "You just love to indulge yourself with dry-curd cottage cheese for lunch and rigorous calisthenics before breakfast." The effect of hypnosis is rarely more than temporary.

"Aversive conditioning" attempts to associate eating with unpleasant events. For example, in one technique the client is told to think about food, then given a slight electric shock, a process that is repeated a number of times. Supposedly, this can help people cut down on eating. However, most individuals simply halt the treatments and resume their usual eating behavior.

I am on a 1,200-calorie weight-loss diet recommended by my doctor. Should I take a vitamin supplement?

Supplements are unnecessary for people following a varied, well-balanced diet of 1,200 calories or more. If you feel more fatigued than usual, you should realize that this is not due to a vitamin deficiency, since vitamins do not provide "pep" or energy. If your total caloric intake and/or carbohydrate consumption is low, and you are not as energetic as usual, you may want to increase your caloric intake by adding bulky carbohydrates, such as whole-grain breads, fruits, and vegetables. Your physician (or a registered dietitian) can advise you further.

I need to lose one hundred pounds. Can a surgical procedure help me?

Any individual who is one hundred or more pounds above the desirable weight range is "morbidly obese," a degree of overweight that is very dangerous. For those aged twenty-five to thirty-five, the death rate is more than ten times greater than it is for their normal-weight peers. Extreme obesity can make it difficult or impossible to exercise. In cases where the overweight condition is threatening the individual's life, a radical approach may have to be considered.

Surgery for weight-loss purposes is indeed a radical approach. The grave risks involved make it a last-choice option, to be selected only after diet/exercise regimens have proven fruitless. The surgical procedures available to the morbidly obese include jaw wiring, intestinal bypass, and gastric stapling.

If a physician advises you to have surgery to avoid premature death from obesity, make sure that you have exhausted all of the other, safer options for achieving weight loss. And do get a second professional opinion.

Can a massage and a sauna at a health club pummel away or evaporate excess fat?

No. Vigorous exercise at a health club (or elsewhere) can help you lose weight—and flab. Massage merely relaxes the muscles; it does not strengthen or firm them, or use up calories (for the person receiving the massage, that is). And don't let the water loss during a sauna fool you. Dehydration causes temporary loss of body fluids— but the lost weight will return as soon as you replenish yourself with a nice cold beverage. Whirlpool baths and jacuzzis also require little exertion, so they do not further weight loss.

Some health clubs and salons provide "passive exercise" machines such as jiggling belts, self-peddling bicycles, moving tables, and rollers that bump over the body. These do nothing to "burn off" calories and lose excess weight. Nor can body wraps, electrical muscle stimulators (EMS), or other gimmicks do anything to improve anyone's weight or body contours.

Can any measures remove cellulite?

"Cellulite" is not a medical term, but was dreamed up at a European diet spa to describe fat deposits on the thighs and buttocks of many overweight and some normal-weight females. These puckery pockets of excess flesh may not disappear with attainment of normal weight.

Cellulite theorists claim that it is composed of a different type of fat, one which contains "toxins" the body has failed to eliminate. However, "cellulite" is just ordinary fat. The orange-peel look is caused by pockets of fat bulging between fibers connecting the skin to underlying tissues. Contrary to advertising hype, neither nutritional supplements nor spot reducers can remove body fat. Mail-order creams claimed to dissolve cellulite typically are lubricating lotions. Some also contain hot pepper or mustard to make the skin tingle, that helps to convince users that the potion is "working." Call it whatever you wish, but remember: the only way to get rid of unwanted poundage is by consuming fewer calories than you expend via a low-calorie diet and a regular program of physical activity.

Does liposuction offer a safe and effective way to improve body contours?

Liposuction is a cosmetic procedure in which fat is sucked out through a small hollow tube inserted into fatty areas of the body. In well trained hands, it has a low complication rate. It is best suited for young adults who wish to rid themselves of fat pockets that persist despite good general weight control. It is theorized that removal of fat cells by liposuction will have permanent results. However, the operation is too new to be certain about its long-term effects.

Can any of the gadgets advertised in magazines help me to lose weight?

If you are referring to "spot-reducing" gadgets, the answer is no. They are all fakes. In fact, even exercises that focus on a single body area will not reduce that area. Unless you lose fat all over through adherence to a successful diet-and-exercise program, exercise will only build up muscles in the exercised area while the fat layer remains the same. Thus, you may "spot-increase" instead of "spot-reduce"! Obviously, a combination of weight reduction and regular exercise is more apt to achieve the results you desire.

Some "spot-reducing" gadgets actually cause fluid loss (through sweating) rather than fat loss, which may result in a temporary reduction in body weight. Heat belts for the waist, body wraps, and rubber sweat suits can cause the wearer to undergo temporary dehydration. They can also prevent sweat from evaporating, which interferes with normal temperature regulation and can be dangerous. Only a vigorous, active workout will help with weight loss. Passive and minimal exercise techniques are ineffective at best.

Your guide to good nutrition

What do you think about the *Fit for Life* Diet?

Fit for Life probably contains more nonsense than any other diet book published in recent years. The authors, Harvey and Marilyn Diamond, hold certificates from the American College of Health Science, a correspondence school that has been ordered by state authorities to stop granting "degrees" or calling itself a college. *Fit for Life* attributes weight gain to eating foods in the wrong combination. According to the Diamonds, this causes the foods to rot in the body so they cannot be assimilated. Toxic wastes then accumulate to cause overweight. To correct this situation they advise eating foods high in water content to "wash the toxic waste from the inside of the body" instead of "clogging" the body. They advise a semi-vegetarian diet in which fats, carbohydrates, and protein foods are eaten at separate meals, with fruit in the morning and vegetables in the afternoon. Computer analysis of their diet has shown it to be marginal in iron and deficient in zinc, calcium, vitamin D, and vitamin B_{12}.

There are so many "diet" books on the market these days. Do authors of such books follow some sort of special format?

Publishers seem willing to publish any diet book that promises to provide a magic answer to the problem of weight control. Books of this type often have the following characteristics:

1. A well known name is used in order to attract attention. The author is a prominent person (outside of the diet/nutrition/health field, of course), or the book is named after a famous place.

2. The services of a ghost writer are used.

3. The title of the book is short and catchy to help it stick in your mind.

4. Miraculous claims are made, such as "lose fat overnight," "eat all you want and still lose weight," or "shed pounds without dieting or exercising." These appeal to the all-American dream of getting something for nothing.

5. Incorrect but scientific-sounding statements, including liberal amounts of half-truths, are peppered throughout the book.

6. The author and/or publisher try to disclaim responsibility by suggesting that a physician be consulted prior to dieting (which is not what most diet book buyers do).

7. The diet itself is nutritionally unbalanced, medically unsound, or even bizarre.

Are any of the current books reliable?

A few are, some of which are listed in Appendix C of this book. To be a savvy consumer, you need to know what to look for and what to avoid. Tables 8:2 and 8:3 summarize our thoughts on common fad diets and sensible alternatives.

Table 8:2. Some Sensible Alternatives

Look for a three-prong approach to weight loss:

1. A well balanced low-fat diet of a wide variety of foods selected from among and within the Basic Four Food Groups
2. A regular program of physical activity
3. Behavior modification for permanent change in lifestyle and eating habits.

Examples of sensible programs include:

1. Individualized programs provided by hospital dietetics departments, university nutrition departments, public health clinics, and physicians and dietitians in private practice
2. Group programs such as Weight Watchers and TOPS
3. Sound diet/fitness books, such as those recommended in Appendix C.

Remember, the only safe and effective method for weight control is the adoption of lifelong health-promoting behavior patterns. By eating a well balanced, low-fat diet and engaging regularly in physical activity, you *can* lose weight and get in shape—for life. Sane eating habits and regular exercise may not be easy at first and won't provide overnight results. But with patience and persistence, you *can* achieve success and enjoy a longer, healthier life.

Table 8:3. Questionable Diet Plans—Past and Present

Diet Plan	Brief Description	Our Comments
Air Force Diet	Low-carbohydrate diet	Unbalanced, causes ketosis and other undesirable side effects; weight loss primarily due to temporary fluid loss
Annapolis Diet	Low-calorie diet with 1 cup of melon at every meal	Unbalanced; low in calcium; can cause slowed metabolism
Atkins Diet	Low-carbohydrate, high-protein diet	Unbalanced, high in fat/cholesterol, causes ketosis and other serious side effects; weight loss primarily due to temporary fluid loss.
Beverly Hills Diet	Fruit for 10 days, gradually adding other foods, but with certain food combinations avoided	Unbalanced, based on myths; serious adverse effects including diarrhea, dehydration, nutrient deficiencies
Bio-Diet	Alternates "crash" diet with binges, plus supplements	Unhealthy practice; supplements do not provide weight-loss benefits as claimed
Bloomingdale's Eat Healthy Diet	Highly restrictive diet based on false premise that certain foods are addictive	Unbalanced, can slow metabolism; semi-starvation encourages binge eating
Calories Don't Count Diet	Low-carbohydrate diet plus safflower oil supplements	Unbalanced, supplements don't provide claimed weight-loss benefits
Diet Center Diet	Low-calorie diet with daily check-ins at Center	Unbalanced, low in calcium, can cause slowed metabolism; expensive

Diet Workshop Diet	Low-calorie diet with group support	Some diet phases are unbalanced and can cause slowed metabolism; group support is helpful to some
Dr. Stillman's Quick Weight-Loss Diet	Low-carbohydrate diet	Unbalanced, cause ketosis and other serious side effects; weight loss primarily due to temporary fluid loss
Drinking Man's Diet	Low-carbohydrate diet	Unbalanced, causes ketosis and other serious side effects; weight loss primarily due to temporary fluid loss
F-Plan Diet	Low-calorie, high-fiber diet	May be deficient in calcium; excessive fiber can cause side effects
Fasting	Juices, teas and/or water only	Dangerous, unbalanced, can slow metabolism
Fat-Destroyer Foods Diet	Low-carbohydrate high-protein diet	Unbalanced, high in fat/cholesterol, causes ketosis and other serious side effects; weight loss primarily due to temporary fluid loss
Fit for Life Diet	Semi-vegetarian, with carbohydrates, fats and proteins eaten at separate meals	Unbalanced; can lead to nutrient deficiencies
Fructose Diet	Low-carbohydrate diet with relatively large intake of fructose	Unbalanced; fructose does not provide weight-loss benefits claimed
Grapefruit Diet	Grapefruit and/or supplements before meals to "burn" fat	Unbalanced and/or ineffective; based on myth

Table 8:3. Questionable Diet Plans—Past and Present (Continued)

Diet Plan	Brief Description	Our Comments
HCG Diet	Very-low-calorie diet plus hormone injections	Unbalanced, can slow metabolism; injections do not provide weight-loss benefits claimed
Herbalife	Very-low-calorie diet plus herbal supplements	Undesirable side effects are common
I Love New York Diet	Alternates "crash" diet with binges	Unhealthy practice, can slow metabolism; promises unrealistic results
Kelp, Lecithin, Vitamin B$_6$ and Cider Vinegar Diet	Low-carbohydrate diet plus supplements	Unbalanced; supplements do not provide weight-loss benefits claimed
Last Chance Diet	Very-low-calorie liquid protein diet	Low-quality protein recommended in book was dangerous and proved fatal.
Liquid protein diets	Formula with low-calorie intake plan	Unbalanced, can slow metabolism; nutrient deficiencies can develop
Mayo Diet	Grapefruit eaten before meals to "bum" fat	Ineffective, based on myth. Not connected with the Mayo Clinic
Mono-food diets	Special emphasis given to one food or food type, such as eggs, grapefruit, or fruit only	Unbalanced; can slow metabolism; nutrient deficiencies can develop
Nutri/System	Prepackaged meals with regular check-ins at clinics	Unbalanced, restrictive; can lead to nutrient deficiencies; expensive

Rice Diet	Five phases, beginning with only rice and fruit	Unbalanced, can cause low blood pressure and lead to nutrient deficiencies
Rotation Diet	Low-calorie diet alternating with "normal" eating	Unbalanced; can slow metabolism; binge eating common
Scarsdale Diet	High-protein diet	Unbalanced, potential for developing ketosis and nutrient deficiencies
Ski Team Diet	Low-carbohydrate diet	Unbalanced, causes ketosis and other serious side effects; weight loss primarily due to temporary fluid loss
Southampton Diet	Low-calorie diet with "mood foods"	Promises unrealistic results, promotes nutrition nonsense
The 35-Plus Diet for Women	Three-phased low-calorie diet for mature women	Unbalanced, restrictive; can slow metabolism
University Diet	Liquid protein diet	Unbalanced, can slow metabolism; nutrient deficiencies can develop
Very-low-calorie diets (protein-sparing modified fasts)	Very-low-calorie diets requiring close medical supervision	Unbalanced, can slow metabolism potentially dangerous, appropriate only for individuals who are at least 30 percent overweight
Any more? Unfortunately, yes. As long as the public buys them, the endless parade of questionable diets will continue.	More of the same	Most likely unbalanced and restrictive and ultimately disappointing; may slow your metabolism and can prove dangerous to your health

9

Healthy Vegetarian Eating

The U.S. Department of Agriculture estimates that some 20 million Americans, about 10 percent of our population, now eliminate meat from their diet. Vegetarian diets have become increasingly popular, mainly for health and economic reasons. With sound nutrition education and some common sense, vegetarians can enjoy a nutritionally adequate diet. It is only when the diet becomes too restrictive and unbalanced that nutrient intake will be inadequate and poor health will result. This chapter provides the dietary facts and sensible guidelines needed to avoid the veggie woes and, if you so choose, to savor a healthy vegetarian diet.

What exactly is a vegetarian diet?

Vegetarians can be classified into five basic groups:

Semi-vegetarian: eats no red meat but does include poultry and fish.

Pisci-vegetarian: eats no red meat or poultry but does include fish.

Lacto-ovo-vegetarian: eats no read meat, poultry, or fish but does include eggs and milk products.

Lacto-vegetarian: eats no meat, poultry, fish, or eggs but does include milk products.

Vegan or *strict vegetarian:* eats *no* animal products.

Some strict vegetarians reject the use of vaccinations because they are prepared from animal cultures, and some refuse to wear shoes or clothing made from animal products—which means no wool, leather, or suede. It is difficult for very strict vegetarians to maintain an adequate diet.

Why do some people choose to be vegetarians?

Diets vary because people have varied tastes, needs, backgrounds, lifestyles, beliefs, and eating habits. The main reasons people choose the vegetarian alternative are: 1) they think it is healthier, 2) they think it is more "natural," 3) they think it is more "ecologic" because it takes less energy to produce vegetarian food than meat, 4) they think it is more economical because of the relatively high cost of meat, and 5) religious dictates. Well known vegetarians of the past include George Bernard Shaw, Leonardo da Vinci, Benjamin Franklin, Voltaire, and Mohandas Gandhi.

Although vegetarianism is still relatively uncommon in this country, Americans have been cutting down on meat consumption during the past decade. At the same time, developing countries have been increasing their meat intake. Many food experts believe that both of these trends are desirable. Increasing the number of farm animals in poorer countries provides protection against famine, because the animals can be slaughtered for food if grain crops fail. Decreasing the number of grazing animals in developed countries enables more crop land to be used to grow food for everyone.

How can one be well nourished on a vegetarian diet?

It is possible to obtain all of the nutrients required for proper growth and health while adhering to a vegetarian diet. However, careful attention must be paid during food selection to ensure that the diet contains adequate supplies of protein, iron, and vitamin B_{12}. If the vegetarian includes milk and milk products, such as yogurt and cheese, plus an occasional egg, nutrient intake should be adequate. This assumes that the rest of the diet is well balanced and includes a variety of fruits, vegetables, grain products, nuts, and legumes (beans and peas).

If milk products are also excluded, it is very difficult to obtain adequate amounts of calcium, phosphorus, riboflavin, and vitamin D. Strict vegetarians who do not take vitamin B_{12} supplements may eventually develop megaloblastic anemia, a serious deficiency disease.

Is it nutritionally unsound to exclude all meat from the diet?

Meat is not essential in the diet for anyone—man, woman, or child—even though it is a nutritious food, which the majority of Americans enjoy. It is an excellent source of protein of the best nutritive quality, of readily absorbable iron, and of other minerals and some vitamins. However, meat is also the main source of fat in the American diet, providing 25 to 50 percent of our total fat intake.

Poultry, fish, eggs, milk, and cheese provide the same high-quality protein and many of the vitamins and minerals found in meat. If the poultry is consumed without the skin, the eggs are not fried, and the dairy products are the low-fat or skimmed variety, fat intake can be kept low. Thus, alternatives to red meat can serve as low-fat substitutes—with some food budget savings to boot.

What foods should be included to ensure a nutritionally adequate vegetarian diet?

Varied selections from the Basic Four Food Groups should be included daily:

1. *Fruit and vegetable group:* all fruits and vegetables, including a citrus fruit daily and a leafy green or bright yellow vegetable every other day.

2. *Grain and cereal group:* whole grain and enriched breads, cereals, pastas, crackers, and other grain products.

3. *Milk and milk products group:* milk, yogurt, cheese, and other foods made with milk. This group is especially important for infants, children, and pregnant and nursing women because milk is the single best dietary source of calcium.

4. *Protein group:* dried beans and peas, lentils, nuts, and eggs.

How can vegetarians obtain adequate protein?

Foods of both animal and vegetable origin provide protein. However, proteins vary in nutritional quality because they differ in the

kinds and amounts of amino acids—the building blocks of protein—
they contain. Meat, fish, poultry, milk, and eggs offer the highest
quality protein because they supply all of the essential amino acids in
the proportions needed by the body. The proteins from some
legumes—particularly soybeans—are close in nutritional quality to
those from animal sources. Combining a small amount of animal protein with plant foods helps to improve the overall protein quality of
one's diet. High-quality protein can also be obtained by consuming
plant foods that are "complementary" in their amino acids—that is,
the amino acids that are insufficient in one food are provided by a
complementing food with an adequate amount. Use the following
combinations to complement plant foods in order to ensure adequate
high-quality protein in your diet:

> *Legumes* plus *grains*
> *Legumes* plus *nuts* and *seeds*
> *Legumes* plus *grains, nuts,* and *seeds*

Table 9:1, which lists foods rich in iron, calcium, riboflavin,
vitamin D, and protein, provides additional guidance for balancing
vegetarian and semi-vegetarian diets.

I find my vegetarian diet is dull
because my main source of protein
is baked beans with wheat bread.
What are some non-animal
sources of protein I might try?

Your diet *does* sound boring! Why not vary it somewhat by using the
complementary protein combinations described above plus a number
of different food choices from the lists below?

Grains: Amaranth, barley, buckwheat, bulgur, corn, kasha
(buckwheat groats), millet, oats, quinoa, rice, sorghum, triticale,
wheat, wild rice,

Legumes: Adzoki beans, anasazi beans, black beans, blackeye
peas (cowpeas), broad beans, chickpeas (garbanzos), kidney beans,
lentils, lima beans, mung beans, navy beans, pea beans, pinto beans,
split peas, soybeans, tempeh, tofu (soybean curd).

Nuts: Almonds, Brazil nuts, cashews, chestnuts, filberts,
pecans, pine nuts, pistachios, tahini, walnuts

Seeds: Poppy seeds, pumpkin seeds, sesame seeds, sunflower
seeds.

Table 9:1. Good Sources of Important Nutrients for Vegetarians and Semi-vegetarians

Iron

Meat, especially organ meats	Dried fruits
Oysters, clams	Dark green leafy vegetables
Dried beans and peas	Potatoes, including sweet potato
Whole grain and enriched breads and cereals	Foods cooked in iron cookware

Calcium

Milk, cheeses	Dark green leafy vegetables
Yogurt	Almonds
Salmon and sardines (with bones)	Soybeans, tofu, fortified soybean milk products

Riboflavin

Milk	Yogurt
Liver	Mushrooms
Cheeses	Enriched grains

Vitamin D

Fish oils	Salmon, sardines
Fortified milk products	Egg yolk
Sunlight	Liver

Protein

Meat, poultry, fish	Dried beans and peas plus nuts and seeds*
Milk, cheese, cottage cheese, yogurt	Dried beans and peas plus grains (barley, corn, oats, rice, rye, wheat)*
Eggs	Peanut butter plus grains*
Soy products (if complete)*	Meat analogs (if complete)*

*A "complete" protein has all the essential amino acids the body requires for proper growth and health. Animal foods provide complete proteins. Plant foods do not, unless eaten in certain combinations (such as those given above) so that the deficiencies in one can be overcome by another.

Do vegetarians have to consume larger quantities of food in order to obtain all the necessary nutrients?

The volume of food required to meet energy and nutrient needs is greater for vegetarians than for individuals on traditional diets. This is because many foods of animal origin are more concentrated sources of energy (higher in fat content) and certain nutrients than are plant foods. Thus, a larger quantity of food may be required in order to fulfill daily requirements. For children and adults with small appetites, this can prove difficult, and undesirable weight loss may result. In such cases, the diet should be carefully restructured to minimize bulky foods and maximize caloric intake. Counseling by a dietitian or other professional nutritionist may be required.

Should vegetarians take vitamin B_{12} supplements?

Vitamin B_{12} is found only in foods of animal origin. Plant foods do not contain any vitamin B_{12}. Therefore, if your diet excludes fish, eggs, milk, and milk products, as well as meat, you should discuss with your physician whether you need vitamin B_{12} supplementation.

Vitamin B_{12} is needed by all cells, particularly those of the nervous system, digestive tract, and bone marrow. Without an adequate supply of vitamin B_{12}, nerve malfunction will occur and growth in children will be stunted. Digestive disturbances, bone marrow maldevelopment, and severe anemia can result. For individuals following restrictive vegetarian regimens, B_{12} supplementation may be essential.

Note: Certain yeasts and meat analogs are fortified with vitamin B_{12}, but be sure to check labels carefully.

Are the synthetic vegetable proteins like TVP (textured vegetable protein) equivalent in quality to the protein found naturally in meat and meat products?

Vegetable protein products are usually fortified with one or more essential amino acids. Fortification raises the protein quality to a level close to that of animal foods. Meat analogs that taste similar to meat are popular protein sources for some vegetarians. When vegetable proteins are added to meat, however (e.g., use of soy protein as a meat extender), missing amino acids are complemented by the meat protein, so the product need not be fortified.

Protein powders are sold in "health food" stores, both as weight-reduction aids and as muscle-building supplements. Such products usually cost much more than equivalent amounts of food containing the same proteins or amino acids. Those that fail to provide complete protein may be dangerous for prolonged use.

What are the disadvantages of a strict vegetarian diet?

The vegan diet excludes all meat, poultry, fish, eggs, milk, and milk products—including cheese and yogurt. This type of diet plan is highly restrictive and can present real health hazards. Protein supplies are often inadequate, and vitamin B_{12} is absent unless supplements are used. Intakes of calcium, riboflavin, vitamin D, and iron may be inadequate as well. All in all, the diet is unbalanced and nutritionally inferior to a nonvegetarian or a more liberal vegetarian diet plan.

Adherence to a strict vegetarian diet is especially dangerous for children and for women who are pregnant or breast-feeding. Adolescents may also find that caloric and nutrient intakes are inadequate for proper growth. A strict vegetarian diet can cause rickets and poor growth in children, inadequate milk supply for nursing mothers, and severe anemia and increased susceptibility to infection at all ages.

What are macrobiotic diets? Are they nutritionally adequate?

Michio Kushi, who founded the Kushi Institute, the Erewhon Natural Foods Company, and the East West Foundation, is the leading proponent of macrobiotics. He characterizes macrobiotics as a "non-religious religion" and a "non-medical medicine" based on "native and intuitive common sense." Kushi Institute literature describes the "standard" macrobiotic diet as follows:

• Whole cereal grains comprise 50–60 percent of each meal. Flour products, noodles and cracked grains, such as unyeasted whole wheat breads, whole wheat and buckwheat noodles, oatmeal, bulgur wheat, cornmeal and other cracked grains may be used to complement main servings of whole cereal grains

- About 5–10 percent of the daily food intake should be soup made with vegetables, seaweed, grains, or beans. Seasonings are usually miso or tamari soy sauce.
- Vegetables comprise 20–30 percent of each meal. Two thirds are cooked; one third may be eaten as raw, pressed salad or pickles. Those for daily use include green cabbage, kale, broccoli, Chinese cabbage, bok choy, dandelion, mustard greens, carrots, squash, scallions, and onions. Potatoes, tomatoes, eggplant, peppers, asparagus, spinach, beets, zucchini, and avocado should be avoided.
- Whole beans or soybean-based products, cooked together with sea vegetables, comprise 5–10 percent of the daily food.
- Beverages include herbal teas, cereal grain teas, spring or well water, and small quantities of fruit juices.
- A small amount of white-meat fish (flounder, carp, halibut, or trout) may be included 1–3 times a week.
- Seasonally available fruit may be eaten 2–3 times a week in small amounts.
- Snacks can include nuts and seeds (dry-roasted and seasoned with sea salt or tamari soy sauce). Popcorn, rice cakes, roasted grains, or beans can also be eaten in small amounts.
- Meat, animal fat, eggs, poultry, milk products, refined sugars, soda, coffee, "chemically treated" foods, refined grains, hot spices, and canned, frozen or irradiated foods should be eliminated.
- Vitamin/mineral supplements are usually avoided, and fluid restriction is common.

The macrobiotic "way of life" includes chewing food at least fifty times per mouthful (or until it becomes liquid), not wearing synthetic or woolen clothing next to the skin, not taking long hot baths or showers (unless too much salt or animal foods has been consumed), having large green plants at home to enrich the oxygen content of the air, and singing a happy song every day.

From a nutrition standpoint, this diet is unnecessarily restrictive. The omission of red meat, eggs, milk, and cheese can result in serious nutritional deficiencies. The elimination of all processed foods is impractical in today's world and could also contribute to dietary deficiencies.

The macrobiotic philosophy promises total health through diet. Yet diet is not the sole cause or cure for all diseases. An unbalanced diet like the macrobiotic regimen is certainly not advantageous to good health. Macrobiotic proponents claim their diet is effective against cancer and AIDS, but there is no scientific evidence behind this claim.

Will a vegetarian diet improve my health?
Can it lower elevated cholesterol levels, help
to decrease high blood pressure, or prevent cancer?

The most effective measure for lowering both blood pressure and blood cholesterol is to reduce body weight to a reasonable level. If you are currently ten, fifteen, twenty, or more pounds over a reasonable or appropriate weight, increased physical activity and a sensible low-calorie diet plan will help to get rid of the excess poundage and may normalize your blood pressure and cholesterol level as well.

It is true that the incidence of high blood pressure, elevated blood cholesterol levels, heart disease, and certain cancers tends to be lower among vegetarians. This may be due in part to the fact that their diet is low in fat and cholesterol and high in fiber, but other lifestyle factors (no cigarette smoking, regular exercise, and moderate alcohol consumption) probably play a role as well. Of course, meat-eaters can—and should—follow these healthful practices too.

Can you summarize the principles of
healthy vegetarian eating?

The best dietary insurance anyone can obtain is a well balanced diet that includes moderate amounts of a variety of foods. Vegetarians can ensure dietary adequacy by following these tips:
- Use whole grain cereals and breads, or choose products that have been fortified or enriched with vitamins and minerals.
- Include legumes of all kinds and combine them with cereals, nuts, and seeds.
- Use fruits and vegetables liberally; they are low in calories and rich in nutrients.
- To supplement a well balanced vegetarian diet beyond any question of adequacy, include dairy products plus occasional eggs.
- If following a strict vegetarian diet, see a physician and/or dietitian for counseling.
- For additional information on vegetarian diets, write to the Department of Nutrition at Loma Linda University, Loma Linda, CA 92354.

As for adopting a vegetarian lifestyle, this is a matter of personal choice. If you do choose this dietary direction—especially a strict vegetarian diet—you may benefit from discussing its nutritional implications with a physician or a registered dietitian.

10

The Truth About Sugar

The American people want sweets. The Government took away cyclamates because of a suggested slight and remote risk of cancer, aspartame (was) held up for years with flimsy evidence of risk, and saccharin remains under attack. Who is going to be in charge—the American people or Big Brother?

This statement ended a letter to the editor that appeared in a prominent newspaper. The writer was pointing out that the value of artificial sweeteners is that they taste sweet—and most people enjoy sweets.

Infants are born with the desire for sweet-tasting things. There is evidence that even the human fetus has a desire for sweet fluids. To most people, the term "sweet" means nice and pleasant, while "sour"and "bitter" can be derogatory terms.

Do Americans eat too much sugar?

Most don't, but food faddists, consumer advocates, and a significant proportion of the general public appear to believe that the average American diet includes large amounts of refined sugar. These claims are made by citing data from the U.S. Department of Agriculture which indicate that Americans use about 132 pounds of caloric sweeteners per year. This number includes all sugars, of which some

61 pounds are sucrose. Most of the rest is fructose from high-fructose corn syrups, which are used extensively in processed foods. These figures actually reflect "disappearance" rather than consumption. But anti-sugar advocates typically refer to the higher number as though it represents sucrose intake.

What is the difference between sweetener consumption and sweetener disappearance?

The difference lies in the amount wasted or used for nonedible purposes and thus not consumed. This includes the granules that stick to the sides of cereal bowls or glasses of iced tea, sugar crumbs that fall off doughnuts and sweet rolls, fermented sugar (used in baking bread or making alcoholic beverages), tray waste in cafeterias, food that goes down the garbage disposal, etc. From the time it is harvested to the time it is consumed, 25 to 30 percent of all food is wasted, including up to 50 percent of vegetables and fruits. Thus sugar consumption rates are considerably lower than sugar disappearance rates. A recent FDA report estimates that sweetener consumption is about 11 percent of total calories.

Another point to consider is that 75 percent of our total sugar intake is consumed as part of other foods. Hence, the nutrients found in the other foodstuffs are consumed along with the sugar. And since we are born with a preference for sweets, we might not even eat certain nutrient-rich foods if they did not contain sugar.

At the present time, there is no evidence to indicate the existence of any health hazard for people who have moderate intakes of sugar. How you satisfy your sweet tooth should be your own choice. This chapter provides the facts on sugar which, together with the information on artificial sweeteners in Chapter 7, will enable you to select your sweets in an informed and responsible manner.

Many people seem to think that sugar is harmful. What are the facts?

Sugar has been unfairly attacked and has received much negative press. This white crystalline sweetening agent has been called "poisonous," "addictive," "empty," "a drug," and even "heroin-like." Sugar has been accused of causing diabetes, heart disease, hypoglycemia, hyperactivity, juvenile delinquency, and even criminal behavior. The truth is that sugar is not poisonous or addictive and that moderate intake is not dangerous. Nor does it cause any of the above problems.

How can we be sure that sugar is safe?

Just think of the chemistry we discuss in Chapter 1. Sugar is pure digestible carbohydrate. Digestible carbohydrates are nutrients and provide calories (energy). All foods that supply energy to the body must be broken down or changed into glucose, the simplest sugar. Thus, table sugar (sucrose), other sugars (such as fructose), all other carbohydrates (starches), and even proteins and fats used for energy are metabolized by the body into glucose.

The fact remains that sugar is one of our most important sources of energy, and the most efficient source of calories in terms of land use. In terms of our ability to produce calories agriculturally, sugar is our least expensive and environmentally soundest source of energy. Sugar is obviously an accessible, efficient, affordable, and tasty source of energy.

Why, then, would anyone attack sugar?

"Health food" promoters typically denounce table sugar while trying to lure consumers into purchasing substitutes at inflated prices. Many unsuspecting consumers have been led to believe that a diet devoid of white sugar is the key to optimal health. They have also been encouraged—by both their own innate desire for sweets and the business tactics of "health food" entrepreneurs—to purchase alternative sweeteners such as "natural" honey, "raw sugar," turbinado sugar, and fructose. The truth is that plain old white sugar is safe, similarly nutritious, and less costly.

Isn't sugar a "junk food"?

As discussed in Chapters 4 and 5, the term "junk food" is as meaningless as the term "health food." All foods contribute to good health when included as part of a varied and well-balanced diet. And any food can be "junky" if eaten to the exclusion of other foods necessary for good nutrition. For example, milk is a nutritious "health food" if a few glasses are included in the daily diet. But if so many glasses of milk are consumed each day that they displace other nutritious foods, the *overall* diet could be unbalanced, nutritionally inadequate, and therefore "junky."

Despite these facts, some consumers feel guilty whenever they eat a candy bar or a slice of pie. A moderate amount of sweets in the diet can be psychologically healthy, since sugar contributes to the enjoyment of eating—and we should eat for pleasure as well as for nutrition. Sweet foods—consumed in moderation—should be called "fun foods," not "junk foods."

Can eating something sweet give you "quick energy"?

Carbohydrates are rapidly digested and absorbed to provide a ready source of energy. So sugar may indeed provide "quick energy." Many "sweets" (such as chocolate candies), though, do contain a significant amount of fat, which is more slowly digested. The best source of "quick energy" is fruit juice, which can provide vitamins and minerals as well.

Does eating too much sugar cause diabetes?

Sugar has never been shown to cause any disease, including diabetes. The main relationship between eating and diabetes is that excess poundage plays a role in the development of diabetes later in life. More than 80 percent of diabetics are over thirty-five and overweight.

Diabetics are advised to balance total food intake in order to attain and maintain a healthy weight. The American Diabetes Association suggests that diabetics limit their intake of total and saturated fat and cholesterol in order to lower blood cholesterol levels and decrease the risk of atherosclerosis.

If diabetes runs in your family, the best advice is to keep your weight at reasonable levels by eating moderately and exercising regularly. Years ago it was thought that once diabetes develops, even small amounts of sucrose would send the blood sugar levels soaring. However, it now appears that most diabetics can handle moderate amounts of sugar without difficulty. If you are diagnosed as diabetic, your doctor can refer you to a registered dietitian to help you plan your diet wisely.

Is fructose better for diabetics than sucrose?

Despite advertisements that promote this concept, fructose should not be used indiscriminately by diabetics or by anyone else attempting to control caloric intake. Fructose is slightly sweeter than sucrose, so a slightly smaller quantity is needed to sweeten foods. However, like sucrose, fructose is converted to glucose in the blood stream, where insulin is needed to metabolize it properly. Thus, fructose does not provide a low-calorie substitute for sugar. And since insulin is still required to complete the metabolism of fructose, diabetics gain little advantage by replacing sucrose with fructose. Diabetics and nondiabetics alike should be aware that purchasing fructose is an overly expensive way to save a few calories.

Does sugar cause hypoglycemia?

True hypoglycemia ("low blood sugar") is rare and is not caused by sugar. If you are troubled by symptoms of fatigue, weakness, shakiness or headaches, your best course of action is to consult a competent physician. For most people, the diagnosis will not prove to be hypoglycemia.

Many food faddists and naive consumers believe that hypoglycemia is a common condition responsible for a whole host of symptoms. Books and magazine articles contribute to the public misconception that sugar-induced hypoglycemia is the culprit responsible for such common symptoms as fatigue, weakness, and headaches. Everyone experiences a temporary decrease in blood sugar, particularly in the morning before breakfast and again 3 to 4 hours after each meal. And a slight drop below normal may occur with improper health habits—lack of sleep, meal skipping, or excessive alcohol intake. Vague symptoms such as fatigue and dizziness are not the typical symptoms of true hypoglycemia, but may be relieved by a glass of juice or a piece of fruit. A diagnosis of hypoglycemia should not be considered unless blood sugar is tested during an attack of symptoms and found to be very low.

Is sugar a factor in the development of heart disease?

A number of dietary factors are related to the development of atherosclerotic heart disease, but sugar does not appear to be one of

them. The amount of total calories, saturated fat, and cholesterol in
the diet are of concern in relation to heart disease (see Chapter 13). In
fact, since high-carbohydrate diets are usually low in cholesterol and
saturated fat, they can help to prevent coronary heart disease. In
1986, a task force assembled by the FDA reported that it had found
no evidence linking sugar intake to cardiovascular disease in the
general population.

Should people who are overweight blame their bulges on "sugar addiction"?

Many Americans who are overweight tend to blame their bulges on
everything—except themselves. Sugar is *not* a physically addictive
substance. The term "addictive" implies that when a substance is
removed from the diet or consumed in smaller amounts, a
"withdrawal reaction" occurs with unpleasant symptoms that can be
relieved by resuming intake of the substance. No evidence exists that
a decrease in dietary sugar causes such a withdrawal reaction.

Overweight is due to a caloric intake that exceeds caloric
expenditure. The cause of obesity is the consumption of excessive
calories, not excessive sugar. Recent evidence suggests that high-fat
diets are more likely than high-carbohydrate diets to produce obesity.

Sustained weight loss requires permanent lifestyle changes,
including regular physical activity and a well-balanced diet (preferably one that is low in fat). Reducing sugar intake without decreasing
total calories and increasing physical activity will not result in weight
loss. Twinkies and cola are far less to blame for the excess flab of
America than are sedentary living habits, overstocked pantries, and
bars!

Then you don't think that sugar causes undesirable behavior?

We certainly don't. Faddists claim that low blood sugar or a diet high
in sugar is a major cause of antisocial behavior. A few school
systems and correctional institutions have eliminated refined sugar
from the food they serve with the hope of improving the behavior of
the populations involved. Perhaps a low-sugar diet can convince
some people to "go straight" to protect themselves from dietary
deprivation, but there is no scientific evidence that eating refined
sugar causes misbehavior. Several well designed experiments have

found no evidence that sugar causes aggressiveness or hyperactivity in children.

What is sugar's role in tooth decay?

Sugar is related to dental caries (cavities), but tooth decay depends not only on the amount of sugar (and other fermentable carbohydrates) consumed, but also the frequency of ingestion and the degree of stickiness. Tooth decay is caused by the dissolving effect on tooth enamel of weak organic acids produced by the bacteria normally present in the mouth. Both sugar and starches provide food for the growth of these bacteria and their acidic by-products. When consumed as part of a meal, sugar is no more cariogenic than starch.

The best advice for avoiding dental decay is to live the first twenty years or so of your life in a community served by fluoridated water. At a level of one part fluoride to one million parts of water, the incidence of tooth decay will be greatly reduced. Regular dental visits are also a must, and good dental hygiene—brushing after meals with fluoridated toothpaste and flossing daily—is important as well.

A well balanced diet with a variety of foods chosen from the Basic Four Food Groups contributes to good oral health. Preferable between-meal snacks are nonsugary foods such as unsweetened yogurt, cheese, raw vegetables, and nuts. Fruit is rich in natural sugars, and dried fruits such as raisins are very sticky and highly cariogenic. The best time to eat sticky sweets is with meals—preferably followed by brushing your teeth or at least rinsing your mouth with water.

The rate of tooth decay has dropped sharply during the past forty years, even though total sweetener consumption has remained unchanged. More than half the children between the ages of five and seventeen have no cavities or other tooth decay. Experts attribute the improvement to the widespread exposure to fluorides and improved levels of oral hygiene.

Would the installation of candy or soft-drink machines in our local high school lead to an increased incidence of tooth decay?

Scientific evidence indicates that frequent consumption of sticky foods containing significant amounts of sugar will result in a higher incidence of tooth decay, especially when such sweets are eaten between meals. However, the sugar in liquids, such as soft drinks and fruit drinks, does not contact the teeth long enough to be a major factor in tooth decay.

Vending machines need not be filled only with candy and soft drinks. They can also be stocked with crackers, nuts, popcorn, milk, yogurt, fresh fruits, and juices. Some students bring a toothbrush to school for use after lunch or snack breaks. But even a quick mouth-rinse at the water fountain after eating can help prevent tooth decay.

Are presweetened cereals a major cause of tooth decay in children?

Several large studies have shown that the rate of tooth decay in children is not influenced by cereals in the diet—whether presweetened or not. About 95 percent of ready-to-eat breakfast cereals are eaten with milk, which significantly lowers their potential for decay. Milk may even protect against tooth decay.

One study, which included over a thousand children, found that those who added table sugar to unsweetened cereals actually consumed more total sugar than those who ate the presweetened types. Many children eat a nutritious breakfast every day because their favorite cereals are available. And since almost all cereals are fortified with vitamins and minerals, a bowl of cereal with milk—plus some orange juice or fruit and a piece of toast—is certainly a nutritious way to start the day.

Are "natural" sweeteners—such as raw sugar, honey, brown sugar, and molasses—more nutritious than regular table sugar?

Many consumers naively assume that the word "natural" on a food label means that the item has not undergone any processing and is free of additives. But this term has no legal definition and is meaningless. "Natural" sweeteners provide a classic example.

"Raw" sugar and turbinado sugar are actually not raw but partially refined to remove impurities. Honey does contain traces of a few minerals and vitamins, but the amounts are so small that their contribution to overall nutrient intake is insignificant. For example, you would have to eat nearly 300 tablespoons of honey in order to obtain the amount of calcium found in a cup of milk. Brown sugar also has trace amounts of some minerals and vitamins but is basically equivalent in nutritional value to white sugar.

Molasses contains larger quantities of several minerals, including iron, calcium, phosphorus, and potassium. For individuals prone to iron deficiency anemia (children and females of childbearing age), the use of molasses as a sweetening agent might be beneficial. However, molasses has a distinctive flavor that some people dislike.

Many manufacturers are using concentrated fruit juice sweeteners in cereals, baked goods, and other products and labeling them "no sugar added, sweetened with natural juices only." Concentrated fruit juice is simply another sweetener and offers no nutritional advantage over ordinary sugar.

The major differences between table sugar and "natural" sweeteners are taste and cost. Purchasing the sweeteners that appeal most to your palate and your budget makes more sense than worrying about their nutrient content.

Sweet foods taste good, so we actually tend to eat a wider variety of foods—including many which add to nutritional status—when our foods are sweetened with sugar. Moderation is the key: a moderate consumption of sugar—like a moderate intake of alcoholic beverages, a moderate amount of daily exercise, and moderation in anything else—can enhance your life and your spirits.

11

Fluid Facts

Food is not our only source of nutritional value and oral satisfaction. Some beverages, too, provide us with energy (calories), various nutrients (particularly water), and refreshment. Drinks replace lost body fluids, quench thirst, and play a significant role in our social activities. After all, what's a coffee klatch without the coffee? Or a social tea without the tea? Or a party without the punch?

As with food, there exist many myths and much confusion about some of our common beverages. Coffee is condemned because of "caffeine phobia"; tea is similarly feared, and the topic of alcohol is surrounded by a multitude of scare stories. Many consumers sip their favorite drink—coffee, tea, beer, or martini—with feelings like those their forebears sixty years ago had when entering a local speakeasy!

Coffee and tea both contain caffeine—as do several other products, including cola beverages, other soft drinks, chocolate, cocoa, some diet pills, and certain headache and cold remedies. Although most of the sensational media stories about the hazards of caffeine are grossly exaggerated, caffeine does exert noteworthy effects on the body. Moderation in intake is thus advisable.

Alcohol, too, exerts druglike effects on the body. Heavy and regular alcohol abuse is accompanied by definite health risks. However, moderate intakes can be consistent with good health. Again, moderation is the answer.

Water is our least expensive thirst-quencher, but the popularity of bottled waters indicates that there is confusion about the best source.

Water is water and, for the price, tap water is usually sufficient and more convenient.

Why is coffee popular?

Coffee has been popular for centuries in many parts of the world. Its distinctive aroma and flavor appeal to many people. In addition, coffee can "perk" people up, help them stay awake, and enhance their endurance and work performance. In this country, the coffee break is common as a means to provide workers with a brief rest and renewed energy. Although coffee is still our most significant source of caffeine, sales have declined in recent years. A National Academy of Sciences committee has reported that the average daily caffeine intake of Americans is the amount contained in two cups of coffee. But much of this caffeine is contained in sodas.

How does caffeine affect the body?

Caffeine can function as a diuretic, a mild antidepressant, an appetite suppressant, and a stimulant. It stimulates the central nervous system and the heart. Caffeine is not stored in body tissues but is metabolized rapidly and efficiently. When ingested, it takes only a few seconds to reach the brain, and a few minutes to enter all other body tissues.

The metabolic effects of caffeine depend on the dosage as well as an individual's tolerance and state of health. The average healthy adult is less sensitive to caffeine than are children and elderly persons. There is also some question about the effect of caffeine intake by pregnant women, since it will cross the placenta, accumulate in the brain of the developing baby, and take twenty to thirty times longer to be eliminated than it does from the adult body. Although tests in laboratory rats have found that a daily dose equivalent to forty cups of coffee can cause fetal abnormalities, there is no evidence that caffeine intake by pregnant women causes birth defects.

Does coffee really provide "pep" and energy?

Coffee consumed without added sugar or cream has only about two calories per cup, but the stimulating effects of caffeine can serve as a quick "picker-upper." Moderate doses can significantly increase work output and lengthen physical performance without affecting motor coordination. Research has also been conducted to determine whether caffeine can enhance athletic performance during endurance events such as long-distance running. So far it appears that ingesting the amount of caffeine in two cups of coffee before an event may improve performance by reserving glycogen (stored glucose) for energy. However, it is unwise to use caffeine for this purpose because it can cause dehydration and intestinal cramps that can hamper performance. Many athletes and coaches regard caffeine as a drug and consider its use unethical.

Will bedtime coffee keep me awake all night?

While some people claim that caffeine does not hamper their sleep, drinking coffee at dinner or bedtime will keep many people awake. Even those who don't notice sleep disturbances may still take longer to fall asleep and may experience a poorer quality of sleep (lighter sleep) when they consume caffeine at bedtime.

What are "coffee nerves"?

The problem of "coffee nerves" may occur in susceptible persons who drink more than four or five cups of brewed coffee per day (or ten to twelve cups of instant coffee, ten to twelve cups of tea, or fifteen 12-ounce cans of caffeinated soft drinks). Sensitive individuals react to smaller amounts. The symptoms include irritability, tremors, poor motor coordination, insomnia, visual disturbances, and a ringing in the ears. Some of these symptoms can be mistaken for anxiety reactions. Chronic excessive coffee consumption can aggravate psychoses in the mentally ill.

Does caffeine bother the digestive tract?

Individuals with certain gastrointestinal problems—such as ulcers or irritable colon—may need to avoid caffeine. It stimulates gastric acid secretions, which can irritate the stomach and can increase contractions of the intestines, which can provoke cramps and diarrhea. There is no evidence that caffeine actually causes ulcers or other gastrointestinal diseases, but it can aggravate any that are present. For some people, even decaffeinated coffee is a gastric irritant.

Some years ago it was speculated that caffeine might cause cancer of the pancreas. Was this confirmed?

Several years ago, a study conducted at Harvard's School of Public Health explored whether coffee ingestion is related to the incidence of cancer of the pancreas. The findings didn't prove that a link exists between the two, but simply suggested that a relationship is possible and indicated that further research is needed. Although the study was preliminary, sensational treatment by the media transformed the results into an exaggerated health scare.

The study was small, the subjects were not in good health, and review by other scientists raised questions concerning the overall design as well as the results of the study. Since the study found that the risk for pancreatic cancer was not elevated in tea drinkers, it is unlikely that caffeine was the carcinogen.

One small study of unhealthy patients is not nearly enough evidence to incriminate caffeine as a carcinogen for healthy individuals. Of course, if you smoke cigarettes during coffee breaks, that is an entirely different story!

Is coffee consumption related to heart disease or stroke?

Between 1986 and 1988, researchers from the Harvard School of Public Health studied more than 51,000 men who were forty to seventy-five years old when the project began. They concluded that total coffee consumption was not associated with an increase in coronary heart disease or stroke.

Does tea contain caffeine?

A pound of tea contains more than a pound of coffee. However, most teas contain about the same amount of caffeine per cup as instant coffee but less than the amount in drip or percolated coffee. Many varieties of noncaffeinated tea are available. The longer a

caffeine-containing tea is steeped, the higher the caffeine content.
Weak tea may be well tolerated by those who need to avoid coffee. If
you drink herbal teas, remember that some contain caffeine or those
other undesirable ingredients noted in Chapter 5. So before buying
herbal teas, read their labels carefully

Table 11:1 illustrates the approximate caffeine content of tea,
coffee, and various other common products.

Table 11:1. Caffeine Content of Foods and Drugs in Milligrams

Coffee (6 oz.)	
Automatic drip	180
Automatic perk	125
Instant	55
Decaffeinated	5
Soft drinks (12 oz.)	
Mountain Dew	55
Mellow Yellow	55
Dr. Pepper	40
Pepsi Cola	40
Coca Cola	35
Tab	30
Tea (6 oz.)	
Iced tea	69
Weak	20-45
Medium	50-60
Strong	70-100
Cocoa	
Chocolate candy (2 oz.)	45
Baking chocolate (1 oz.)	45
Milk chocolate candy (2 oz.)	10
Cocoa powder (6 oz.)	10
Drugs (per capsule or tablet)	
Dexatrim	200
Nodoz	100
Anacin	32.5
Midol	32.4
Coricidin	30

Do alcoholic beverages offer any nutritional value?

Alcoholic beverages were used in ancient times for nourishment as well as for religious and social purposes. Modern alcoholic beverages are virtually devoid of nutrients and are not used extensively for religious purposes. But these beverages still play a significant role in social and cultural functions and are used for relaxation by millions of Americans.

Most alcoholic beverages are high in calories, and all have negligible nutritional value (except for drinks made with nutritious mixers such as fruit juice). Some "light" beers and wines contain fewer calories than the standard beers and sweeter wines.

What does "proof" mean? Is it related to caloric value?

The alcoholic content of distilled spirits—gin, vodka, bourbon, and scotch—is expressed in terms of "proof." In this country, the proof represents twice the alcohol content by volume. Thus, "100-proof" means 50 percent alcohol, and "80-proof" is 40 percent alcohol. Most liqueurs range from 40 to 55 percent alcohol content.

The alcohol content of wines and beers is expressed as a percentage of volume. White table wines usually contain 9 to 12 percent alcohol by volume, red wines up to 14 percent, and fortified wines have 20 to 24 percent due to addition of extra alcohol. Wine coolers range from 4 to 6 percent, or even more, depending on the brand. Beer—including ales, lagers, and stout—can contain anywhere between 3 and 8 percent alcohol, with "light" beers at the lower end of the spectrum.

The non-alcohol balance of an alcoholic beverage consists mainly of water. Beer and wine contain some carbohydrate, especially the darker beers and sweeter wines. Some alcoholic beverages—particularly bourbon and others with a dark color—also contain small amounts of congeners, substances that impart the characteristic flavor. Congeners are also believed to add to the aftereffects of alcohol use known as "hangovers."

A simple formula for determining the caloric contents of an alcoholic beverage (without mixer) is: calories = 0.8 x proof x ounces. The higher the proof, the greater the number of calories. Remember, however, that beer is usually consumed in 12-ounce servings, wine is sipped in 3- or 4-ounce glasses, and the typical "hard" drink is made with an ounce or two of the alcoholic beverage. So the calories in the lower-proof beverages can add up faster than many people realize.

Tables 11:2 and 11:3 depict the alcohol and caloric content of common alcoholic beverages and mixers.

Table 11:2
Caloric Content of Alcoholic Beverages

Beverage	Proof or % Alcohol	Amount (Oz.)	Calories (Approx.)
Liquor, distilled	80 proof	1.5	95
	86 proof	1.5	105
	90 proof	1.5	115
	100 proof	1.5	125
Beer, "light"	3.2%	12	95
Beer, regular	4.5%	12	150
Ale	5%	12	165
Wine, cooler	3%	6	150
Wine, table	12%	3.5	90
Wine, fortified (sherry, port)	19%	1.5	140

Table 11:3
Caloric Content of Mixers

Mixer, 6 Ounces	Calories (Approx.)
Club soda	0
Tonic	55
Collins	60
Ginger ale	60
Seven-up	75
Cola	75
Fruit punch	80
Bitter lemon	85
Cranberry cocktail	110
Eggnog	225
Cream	385

If alcohol is high in calories,
why are many alcoholics underweight?

The main reason alcoholics lose weight is that alcohol depresses their appetite for food. Also, alcohol does not provide the body with energy in the same way other foods do. Alcohol yields about seven calories per gram, while carbohydrate provides only four. Yet laboratory studies show that there is somewhat less weight gain with alcohol than with calorically equivalent amounts of carbohydrate. Substituting alcohol for carbohydrate for half the total calories in an otherwise balanced diet results in weight loss. Many of the calories provided by alcohol appear to be dissipated by the body as heat (hence the warm flush that accompanies indulgence). Eventually, alcohol abuse interferes with normal digestion and metabolism so that the body is unable to properly use the nutrients that are consumed.

Is it smarter to drink beer or wine
rather than hard drinks?

It is smartest to limit total consumption, no matter what you choose to drink. Some people believe that they are automatically consuming less alcohol if they drink wine or beer rather than distilled liquor. But alcohol is alcohol, whether in beer, wine, or martinis. It's the quantity of alcohol consumed, not the type of beverage, that is important.

Moderation in the consumption of all alcoholic beverages is wisest. And if you are watching your waistline, the "light" beers or "light" wines are relatively low-calorie choices—unless, of course, you drink twice as much.

What health damages can alcohol abuse cause?

Unlike foods, most alcohol is absorbed from the stomach directly into the blood stream. The rate of absorption depends on individual size and metabolism, the speed of alcohol consumption, and the presence of food in the stomach. If alcohol is imbibed faster than it can be metabolized, it accumulates in the blood and body tissues, causing the symptoms of drunkenness. Most adults cannot consume more than one ounce of alcohol per hour (approximately two "drinks") without exhibiting physical and/or psychological side effects.

Since alcohol is metabolized by the liver, long-term heavy consumption may damage this organ, causing scarring (cirrhosis), which interferes with its normal functioning. About 10 percent of heavy drinkers develop this condition. Alcohol abuse can also cause stomach irritation (gastritis), reduced immunity to illness, nutrient deficiencies (when decreased appetite leads to inadequate intake of food), and a host of other health problems.

Can alcohol cause cancer?

Heavy drinkers who smoke cigarettes have an increased risk of developing cancer of the esophagus or oral cavity. For example, a two-pack-a-day cigarette smoker has more than double the risk than a nonsmoker of developing cancer of the oral cavity. If two alcoholic drinks are also consumed each day, the risk is increased fifteen-fold.

Press reports have stated that whiskey and beer cause cancer. Is this true?

Several studies have found small amounts of nitrosamines (formed during the process of barley malting) in certain brands of Scotch whiskey and beer. Large doses of nitrosamines may cause cancer in animals. However, the effect of nitrosamine intake on humans—if any—is questionable. No human case of cancer has ever been correlated with the consumption of nitrosamines (see Chapter 7).

The finding of nitrosamines in these particular alcoholic beverages led the beverage industry to alter its processing methods to reduce the quantities of these compounds in Scotch whiskey and beer.

What about urethane, the chemical that forms during fermentation of certain beverages?

The risks associated with the consumption of urethane are unknown. Studies with various experimental animals indicate that this chemical—a byproduct of fermentation—may be carcinogenic in far larger doses than are consumed by humans. The FDA and the Bureau of Alcohol, Tobacco, and Firearms have been sampling alcoholic beverages to determine the average levels of urethane in products currently available to consumers. The National Toxicological Program is studying the risk this chemical poses in alcoholic beverages. Meanwhile, due to public concern, the beverage industry has voluntarily reduced urethane levels in American-made wines and whiskeys.

Can lifelong alcohol intake patterns affect the chances for developing heart disease?

Cardiomyopathy, a disease in which the major heart muscle is weakened, occurs more frequently in heavy drinkers than in nondrinkers. However, the more common forms of heart disease in this country are not caused by alcohol intake. In fact, the incidence of coronary heart disease is somewhat lower among moderate drinkers than among abstainers and former drinkers. The reason for this is unclear, but it may be because moderate intake of alcohol increases the amount of HDL ("good cholesterol") in the blood.

Will alcohol intake during pregnancy have any effect on the developing baby?

Like many other drugs, alcohol passes through the placenta and into the blood stream of the fetus. An excessive fetal intake of alcohol can have disastrous consequences. Although there is no evidence that an intake of one ounce a day is harmful to the fetus, most health professionals recommend abstinence during pregnancy to be on the safe side. Unfortunately, most women don't know they are pregnant during the first few weeks after conception.

Fetal alcohol syndrome (FAS) is a combination of birth defects in babies born to women who drink excessively during pregnancy. FAS babies are abnormally small at birth. Unlike other small newborns, they seldom catch up to normal growth. Most exhibit some degree of mental deficiency and appear jittery and poorly coordinated. Almost half have heart defects, and all have malformed facial features: narrowed eyes, a low nasal bridge, and a short, upturned nose.

Over one million women of childbearing age are alcoholics—and the incidence is increasing, particularly among adolescents. Fetal alcohol syndrome is a tragedy, but a preventable one. All women of childbearing age can prevent the birth defects caused by excessive use of alcohol. Additional information on this subject can be provided by the March of Dimes Birth Defects Foundation, 1275 Mamaroneck Avenue, White Plains, NY 10605; or the National Maternal and Childbearing Clearinghouse, 3520 Prospect Street, N.W., Washington, DC 20057.

Can you say how much alcohol is safe?

For most people, a moderate intake of their favorite cocktail—that is, one or two drinks—can be enjoyable, sociable, and fun. Alcohol can be included in a well balanced diet as long as it doesn't take the place of foods essential to good health. Of course, for anyone who plans to get behind the wheel of a car, abstinence is always the safest policy.

Is there any advantage to drinking bottled water instead of tap water?

In most communities, there is no significant health advantage to drinking bottled water. Tap water is usually acceptable and always less expensive. But bottled waters, both carbonated and uncarbonated, are growing in popularity as an alternative to alcoholic beverages. If you want a noncaloric substitute for your favorite cocktail, try a cold glass of water, with a twist of lemon—guaranteed to be hangover-free.

Does water softness or hardness have any effect on health?

"Hard" water contains various amounts of calcium and magnesium that many people find bothersome. (Soaps do not lather as well in hard water, and mineral deposits can interfere with the functioning of various home appliances.) When water is "softened," most of the calcium and magnesium are replaced by sodium. Studies conducted in the U.S. and Canada show that death rates from cardiovascular disease may be as much as 15 to 20 percent higher for populations using soft water than for those using hard water.

Significant amounts of sodium are added to water by the softening process. Most city water supplies have less than 20 mg of sodium per liter. Softening may raise this to 75 mg per liter, an undesirable level for individuals who must restrict sodium intake for medical reasons. Such individuals may find it useful to obtain bottled water that is sodium-free or contains very little sodium. People who wish to enjoy the convenience of soft water but retain the possible health advantages of drinking hard water can use a water softener but bypass it with one pipe to the cold water tap in their kitchen.

I hear there is a new hormone that can boost milk production in cows. Does it pose any risks?

Bovine somatotropin (BST) can boost the milk output of cows by about 15 percent. BST is produced naturally in the anterior pituitary gland of cattle. Using recombinant DNA technology, scientists have been able to make it at a price low enough for commercial use.

Milk produced by BST-treated cows is no different from milk produced by untreated cows. Because lactating cows produce BST naturally, small amounts are found in the milk of untreated cows. BST treatment does not increase these levels. Regardless, BST is a protein that is digested like any other protein in milk and is not biologically active when ingested by humans. In other words, BST can produce the same milk at lower cost without the slightest risk to consumers.

A final comment

People often overlook fluids in considering their nutritional intake, but beverages are an important component of our overall diet. The caloric and nutrient contributions of our favorite fluids should be taken into account whenever taking a coffee break, attending a party, or simply reaching for a thirst quencher. Fruit and vegetable juices, low-fat milk and yogurt drinks, or just plain water can add nutrients to the diet without piling on the calories. Variety in beverage choice, as in food selection, is an important aspect of balancing the diet.

Both caffeine and alcohol have druglike effects that, in excess, can be detrimental to health. Common sense and self-control in the consumption of coffee, tea, colas, beer, wine, and liquor are the keys to safe use. In moderation, such beverages can impart pleasure and satisfaction. In excess, they can jeopardize your health. Such decisions are your own responsibility.

12

Tips for Teenagers

There are a several reasons to be concerned about the eating habits of teenagers. First, since the growth spurts preceding sexual maturation require more nutrients for the body than at any other time (except during pregnancy and lactation), nutritional demands during this age span are very high. Second, adolescence is a time for casting off old habits and trying on new identities—which often means that dietary advice given by adults is rejected. Third, teens are very susceptible to fads, including fad diets, some of which pose serious threats to health. Since habits formed during adolescence frequently continue into adulthood, it is good for teenagers to become accustomed to following a well balanced diet.

This chapter emphasizes two diet-related problems of adolescence. The first is anorexia nervosa, a disorder whose victims starve themselves into states of emaciation, malnutrition, and even death. The second problem is meeting the nutritional needs of athletes. Sports and fitness activities often increase teenage vulnerability to nutrition myths, fad diets, and unnecessary food supplements.

My 15-year-old daughter has only a bit of baby fat to lose but thinks she needs a drastic diet. What can I do?

Fad diets limited to one or two types of food, or which eliminate an entire food group, inevitably exclude some essential nutrients as well. Remind your daughter that she is still growing and requires a well balanced diet in order to function properly and reach her potential for height, bone structure, and feminine shape.

Eating moderately and exercising regularly is the best method for losing weight and the safest. Many young girls who adopt crash diets go to extremes, losing too much weight and jeopardizing their health. Loss of "baby fat" is best achieved by selecting a variety of foods from the Basic Four Food Groups but using smaller-than-usual portion sizes (particularly of meats and whole milk products), cutting down on high-calorie snacks and desserts, and becoming more physically active. If your daughter is "turned off" by your advice, she might benefit from seeing a registered dietitian or other professional for diet counseling.

I am in high school and know I should lose weight, but I just can't seem to do it. Will skipping breakfast every day or eliminating lunch help me lose weight?

You may lose weight initially, but starving yourself will also produce feelings of deprivation, hunger, and frustration that will eventually lead to overindulgence. Why torture yourself with a growling, empty stomach that constantly reminds you of how hungry you are, tempts you to snack on all the wrong things, and makes you so uncomfortable by dinner time that you end up pigging out? The body is like a race car—it needs regular refueling. The best plan for smooth functioning—and no "engine" trouble—is to refuel at regular intervals during the day without overloading the tank. Get out there and move around, too!

Meal-skipping is a common practice in our fast-paced society, especially among on-the-go teens. Yet such drastic dietary alternations can lead to abnormal eating patterns, excessive weight loss, and poor health. Establishing healthy eating habits during your teen years can help you avoid ill effects later on. Besides, you'll be a lot happier and easier to get along with if you eat sensibly than if you're constantly hungry and ready to bite everyone's head off.

My 17-year-old daughter is painfully thin. How can she gain some weight?

While much attention has been focused on the problems of people who need to lose weight, there are a significant number of people at the other end of the spectrum who also deserve consideration. Being "painfully" thin may not only hurt one aesthetically; it can also be a definite health hazard. Severely underweight people (20 percent or more below reasonable weight) are more susceptible to illness and may lack physical endurance, tire easily, and have trouble concentrating. Also, when body fat is too low, menstruation may be irregular.

Gaining weight is as difficult for some people as shedding extra pounds is for others—particularly during adolescence, when body energy requirements are high. To gain weight, extra calories must be taken in. For some people, simply eating larger amounts at mealtimes works best. For others, the answer is between-meal snacks in addition to regular meals, but eaten one or two hours beforehand so as not to dull the appetite for the upcoming meal. Mild physical activity can help to increase appetite, as can looking at pictures of appetizing foods and inhaling tempting food aromas. Muscle-building exercise can also put on pounds—as shapely muscles instead of undesirable excess fat.

What is anorexia nervosa? My teenage daughter has dieted—really starved herself—to below 100 pounds, so I'm afraid she may have this disorder.

In our weight-obsessed society, eating disorders have become epidemic. During the past decade, anorexia has been documented with such increased frequency that it has become a prominent topic in the media. Often described as "the relentless pursuit of excessive thinness," the condition occurs predominantly in young women. Although anorexia nervosa is not a new problem and was described more than a hundred years ago, recognition of its underlying psychosocial causes is a relatively recent development. If untreated, anorexia nervosa can prove fatal. Since most anorectics (over 90 percent) are female, the discussion in this chapter applies primarily to females.

Self-starvation may begin with a simple reducing diet, pursued with excessive zeal and a determination to excel that are characteristic of the anorectic personality. For the individual who feels inadequate, a new sense of power may accompany weight loss. The feeling of power and pride increases as more weight is lost and the anorectic feels in control—of her own body.

Anorectics typically starve themselves into a "concentration camp" appearance, indulge in strenuous activity, but insist that they are neither hungry nor tired. Yet they tend to be preoccupied with food and often become bulimic. (Bulimics "binge and purge"—gorge themselves, then induce vomiting and use diuretics and/or laxatives.) Many anorectics undergo a personality transformation, becoming surly, secretive, and uncooperative.

Bulimia without anorexia is also on the rise. Its health detriments can be severe, and its victims often need psychological as well as dietary counseling.

If your daughter is starving herself, losing weight, and refusing to admit to her dieting obsession, you should get professional help for her—both medical and psychological. Anorexia nervosa can lead to chronic malnutrition, which results in biological changes that influence the victim's thinking, behavior, and feelings. It may be a struggle to convince your daughter that she needs help, but her health—and life—may depend on it.

What social and psychological factors are related to anorexia nervosa?

A number of case histories were documented by the late Dr. Hilde Bruch, a psychiatry professor who was one of the world's leading authorities on eating disorders. Her book *The Golden Cage: The Enigma of Anorexia Nervosa* cited the following psychosocial characteristics common to anorectics:

• They come from upper- or upper-middle class homes with an apparently harmonious, well organized family life; the few who come from lower- or middle-class homes have families that are upwardly mobile and success-oriented. Child-raising practices have been carried out by extremely conscientious mothers, with both parents showing a tendency to determine not only the child's behavior, but *all* activity, thought, and desire. A great deal is expected of the child.

• Until the onset of their condition, anorectics typically are described as "model" children by parents, teachers, friends, and neighbors. They are obedient, considerate, dependable, even-tempered. They usually excel in schoolwork and are rather shy.

• When treatment enables them to express their inner thoughts, they reveal feelings of never-quite-measuring-up to expectations, not being good enough, and not being worthy of privileges. They also express fear of not being loved, and may have no sense of personal accomplishment.

• Often they perceive themselves as mere puppets, whereby their own achievements are really only their parents' achievements. Many anorectics often have no sense of their own goals. They may have great difficulty in making decisions and have a chameleonlike tendency to take on the personalities of their associates.

• Any number of fears or frustrations may trigger a policy of self-starvation. Common triggers—all of which involve fears of maturation—include separation from home, attention from the opposite sex, and loss of girlfriends to boys.

How can anorexia nervosa be treated?

This condition requires psychological and dietary counseling as well as medical treatment for any physical ailments that have developed. It is essential that medical and psychological therapy be provided simultaneously, since the patient's malnutrition can alter normal thinking processes. Separating the anorectic temporarily from the dynamics of home life may be helpful. If the patient's weight is dangerously low, hospitalization with intensive therapy is usually recommended. Medical treatment may have to include tube feedings or hyperalimentation (complete nutrition through the veins) if the patient will not or cannot eat. Dietary counseling may help the anorectic understand the importance of nutrition and instill healthy eating behaviors. Psychological therapy should guide her toward greater self-understanding, clarification of family dynamics, and the development of her own individual personality. At the conclusion of successful treatment, she should at least be approaching a healthy weight range and be motivated to maintain a reasonable weight. And she should also be able to feel "special" and proud—for the right reasons instead of the wrong ones.

If we know how to treat eating disorders, why are they on the rise?

Anorexia and bulimia are being stimulated by our society's preoccupation with body image and dieting. These disorders often take root during adolescence, when teens are more concerned with their looks than with their health. Most teenagers are worried about gaining undesirable weight, and many girls of normal weight consider themselves fat. A recent study found that 75 percent of female teens perceived themselves as overweight, nearly 40 percent were dieting, and more than 20 percent weighed themselves obsessively. Reasons for this preoccupation with body weight include:

1. Current fashion trends favor the thin look.

2. Even if they don't need to lose weight, daughters will often identify with their diet-conscious mothers.

3. More girls are becoming involved in athletic activities for which leanness is advantageous.

4. During puberty, body fat is distributed onto the hips, thighs, and breasts of growing girls, who may then embark on a campaign to rid themselves of these normal fat deposits.

Dieting can also be a source of conversation, a means for attracting attention, or a kind of game in which teens try out various fad diets. Some preteens and teenagers have permanently stunted their growth by self-imposed starvation during the time when they should be undergoing their growth spurt—a condition called "nutritional dwarfism." Yet it is unlikely that the eating disorder epidemic will diminish unless our society shifts emphasis from leanness-at-any-cost to health-for-health's-sake.

My son is on the high school wrestling team. Before almost every match, he goes on a starvation diet so he can meet his weight. Afterward he pigs out. Doesn't this pattern pose nutritional hazards?

When "making weight" involves starvation and binges, performance may be hampered and nutritional status jeopardized. Weight-obsessed wrestlers may also become dehydrated, which is dangerous. The best body weight for competition in any sport is at the level that allows for proper hydration and optimal musculature without extra body fat. Starving before a competition will only serve to weaken your son and stunt his growth. Your son—and his coach—should be aware that such dietary habits can cause detrimental physical and psychological effects. "Yo-yo dieting" can also make weight control more difficult in the long run. A recent study of twenty-seven adolescent wrestlers found that the resting metabolic rate and resting energy expenditure of those who repeatedly lost and regained weight were lowered.

By informing your son that crash dieting may interfere with his growth, you may persuade him to try the safer, more conventional means for weight control. When he finds that a well balanced diet actually aids his performance, watch out that he doesn't hurt you—with a big bear hug.

My son, a high school track participant, seems be running himself thin. He claims that all athletes have less body fat and therefore weigh less. Is there any way to find out whether he is unhealthfully thin?

Athletes generally do have more muscle and less fat, but muscle actually weighs more than fat. Runners are usually quite lean, but your son can jeopardize his health—and performance—by losing too much weight. A sports medicine specialist can perform various tests, such as skin-fold measurements, to determine your son's current body fat percentage and a desirable weight. A visit with a registered dietitian or sports nutrition professional can give both of you the facts to prevent further worrying and protect your son's health.

Do athletes have special nutritional needs?

The nutritional requirements of athletes are actually similar to those of sedentary individuals. Training increases the need for calories, since exercise uses them up. This need can be met by increasing portion sizes at meals and snacking in between.

Fluids lost during exercise need to be replaced, and water is the best choice. Fruit and juices can also help to quench thirst, as can the more costly "athletic drinks." Alcoholic beverages, including beer, are not a good choice, since they act as diuretics and tend to deplete the body of fluids. Colas, coffee, and tea contain caffeine, which can also act as a diuretic.

Although there is no magic diet for athletes, performance can be impaired if one's diet is inadequate. The best diet for any athlete is one that he or she enjoys and which also provides a variety of nutritious foods and fluids in amounts adequate to maintain desirable weight and support optimal performance.

Do athletes require more protein than non-athletes?

Individuals engaged in strenuous athletics may need a bit more protein than their sedentary peers. However, since athletes tend to eat more food, following the Basic Four Food Group system will ensure an adequate protein intake, even during rigorous training periods. Actually, most Americans consume at least twice as much protein as they need.

Today's "training table" is more apt to be stocked with energy-fueling carbohydrates—such as bread, potatoes, pasta, cereal, and fruit—rather than the high-fat steak-and-eggs of the past. For athletes in training, the ideal diet contains 12 to 15 percent of total calories as protein, about 30 percent as fat, and the rest as carbohydrates. Protein supplements are unnecessary, expensive, and potentially harmful.

Are candy bars a good afterschool snack to eat for "quick energy" before sports practice?

Candy bars, which are high in sugar, can provide a quick source of energy. However, it is best not to eat anything for at least two hours prior to strenuous exercise, and to keep the pre-activity meal light.

What is "carbohydrate loading"?

Endurance during prolonged exercise can be enhanced by "carbohydrate loading" to increase the glycogen (stored energy) content of the liver and muscles. Sports nutrition specialists now recommend a milder program than in the past, because drastic dietary deviations can cause discomfort and, if repeated too often, ill health. The current prescription is to increase carbohydrate to 70 percent of total calories during the week before an endurance event. In large amounts, carbohydrate can increase the glycogen stores of the liver and muscles, which will provide additional fuel during prolonged exercise. The best sources are complex carbohydrates such as pasta, potatoes, dried beans, breads, and cereals. Note that carbohydrate loading is only effective when training for endurance events such as marathons and triathlons.

Do athletes need vitamin or mineral supplements?

No! Nutritional supplements—vitamins, minerals, and special "athletic packs"—should not be self-prescribed by athletes or any healthy person consuming a well-balanced diet. For elite runners, the threat of iron deficiency requires monitoring by a sports medicine professional who will prescribe supplements only if needed. There is no magic food or supplement that can add to athletic performance. What counts most is proper training!

Should athletes take salt pills?

No. Any sodium lost with perspiration is easily replaced with moderate use of the salt shaker. Salt tablets can cause gastric upset and can actually lead to dehydration.

Bodybuilding magazines are loaded with ads for amino acid combinations that supposedly help build muscles and increase endurance. Are they effective?

No. Protein needs are easily met during weight training by eating a well balanced diet, which will supply all the amino acids needed for muscle-building. Unbalanced amino acid combinations do not build muscles and may lead to ill health. Beware of advertisements that promote diet aids as if they were drugs. Some of them are claimed to be "steroid substitutes" or "growth hormone releasers." These claims—which are based on fanciful interpretations of animal experiments—are both false and illegal.

A good diet plus proper training will help build muscles and endurance—safely, effectively, and in the proper manner of a "good sport." Steroid drugs may enhance these effects in some individuals, but they are not safe. Athletes who use large doses can damage their body permanently or experience temporary complications that last for months after the drug is stopped. The problems include testicular atrophy, pituitary inhibition, prostate enlargement, fluid retention, high blood pressure, kidney damage, acne, fibrosis of the liver, breast enlargement (in both sexes), and unwanted hair growth (in women). Some athletes have even died as a result of steroid use.

Unfortunately, the application of nutrition to sports medicine and physical fitness—like so many other areas of health—has been fraught with misinformation and myths. There are no magic foods that lead to super power or agility. Nutritional supplements serve mainly to supplement the profits of those who manufacture and sell them. Dietary deficiencies can affect performance, but food fads and supplementation by a well nourished athlete will not improve ability and may even result in ill health. It is safer, cheaper, and wiser to simply eat a well balanced diet selected from among and within the Basic Four Food Groups. Eating wisely—plus regular physical activity—can keep nutritional status high and weight at a desirable level in preparation for a healthy adulthood.

13

Diet, Heart Disease, and Cancer

Heart disease and cancer are two of our country's leading causes of death and disability. During recent years, a great deal of scientific research and public attention have focused on the prevention of these conditions. Based on current evidence, faulty diet is implicated as an underlying factor for the common types of heart disease and several types of cancer. This chapter provides the information you need to reduce your odds of developing these conditions.

Can changes in dietary habits reduce the incidence of heart disease?

Cardiovascular disease is the leading cause of death in this country, claiming more than 900,000 lives each year. Coronary heart disease (CHD) is the major cardiovascular disease and accounts for about half of this total. The death rate from heart disease has decreased considerably during the last three decades. This reduction is related to changes in our dietary patterns, as well as to four other factors: many adults have stopped smoking; many have increased their physical activity; high blood pressure is now diagnosed earlier and treated more effectively; and emergency care for heart attacks has improved. The beneficial dietary changes have included lowering the intakes of total calories, saturated fat, and cholesterol.

What causes CHD?

CHD is the most common cause of heart disease. It is caused by atherosclerosis, which leads to narrowing of the arteries that nourish the heart (coronary arteries). If a narrowed blood vessel is suddenly blocked by a blood clot, the area of the heart just beyond the blockage is denied oxygen and nourishment, resulting in a "heart attack" (myocardial infarction). The situation often is complicated by the development of an irregular heart rhythm and/or reduction of the heart's power to pump blood.

What causes atherosclerosis?

Like other chronic degenerative diseases, atherosclerosis can take years to develop. The gradual thickening of artery walls may be due to:
   • Arterial damage from build-up of fatty substances and cholesterol
   • Repeated injury to arterial walls
   • Chemical changes that transform the normal lining cells into benign tumor cells
   • Viral infections.
   Diet is implicated in atherosclerosis because the deposits on arterial walls contain high levels of fat and cholesterol. Studies of both humans and animals have shown links between dietary habits and atherosclerosis.

What is cholesterol?

Cholesterol is a waxy, fatlike substance found only in animal cells. It is made in several body tissues, particularly the liver, and is present in all foods of animal origin and none of vegetable origin. Cholesterol is essential for proper body function, aiding in the formation of vitamin D, certain sex hormones, bile acids, and all cell membranes.
   The amount of cholesterol in the diet can affect blood cholesterol levels, although the amounts of saturated fat and total calories are more significant. Egg yolks and organ meats (liver, kidney, sweetbreads) are high in cholesterol. Fatty meats, butter, cream,

whole milk, and most cheeses also contain cholesterol, but much less than is present in egg yolk.

Does cholesterol cause CHD?

Cholesterol alone is not the cause of heart disease. An elevation in the blood level of cholesterol increases the likelihood of heart disease. However, CHD is a multifactorial disease. Risk factors include heredity, being male, age, high blood pressure, cigarette smoking, lack of physical activity, obesity, diabetes, and stress, as well as elevated blood cholesterol. The more risk factors you have, the greater your risk of heart disease. Heredity, gender, and age cannot be controlled, but the other risk factors can be influenced.

How do blood lipoproteins fit into the risk-factor picture?

Lipoproteins are compounds of fat and protein that are typed according to their density. Studies indicate that high-density lipoproteins (HDL) may help to prevent heart disease, while the low-density forms (LDL) are a serious risk factor in CHD. HDL appears to help remove cholesterol from the artery walls and may also impede the arterial damage caused by LDL.

The Framingham Heart Study, a research project spanning some 40 years and funded by the National Heart, Lung, and Blood Institute, found that individuals with low levels of HDL have many times the incidence of heart disease as do persons with high HDL levels. This finding has been confirmed by several other studies. The following data have also been disclosed:

• Women of reproductive age have 30 to 60 percent more HDL and a much lower rate of CHD than males.

• The HDL levels in dogs and rats are high, and these species are quite resistant to atherosclerosis.

• Individuals with diabetes, obesity, and hypertension all have low levels of HDL and a high incidence of heart disease.

For many people, a diet low in calories, saturated fat, and cholesterol will decrease *total* blood cholesterol and increase HDL. Regular exercise may exert the same effects. Your goal should be to maintain a reasonable blood cholesterol level, with the "good" HDL high and the "bad" LDL low. Laboratories that determine total cholesterol can also determine your HDL and LDL levels.

What level of blood cholesterol is considered "elevated"?

This is difficult to answer precisely, because there is some disagreement among experts about which levels warrant aggressive action. However, the levels regarded as "normal" have decreased during the past several years. Most medical authorities now consider any level above 240 mg of total cholesterol as high and consider 180 to 220 as an acceptable range. The National Cholesterol Education Program recommends that adults whose total cholesterol level is 200 or above have additional tests to determine their levels of LDL and HDL and discuss the findings with a physician.

What are doctors likely to recommend?

Treatment recommendations are based primarily on LDL levels. If the LDL level is 130 or above, the patient usually is advised to begin a diet that is no greater than 30 percent fat. If the patient also is overweight, weight reduction is advised too. However, if the LDL is extremely high (greater than 225) or the patient has definite CHD, a stricter diet or drug therapy may be initiated. Weight control, regular exercise, and smoking cessation are also essential for people who wish to lower their risk of heart attacks. Very low HDL levels (under 35) may also indicate a need for medical intervention.

Should all adults be concerned about the fat content of their diet?

Most authorities recommend that overall fat consumption be limited to about a third of the total caloric intake, with an emphasis on unsaturated fats. This means consuming lower quantities of animal foods that are high in saturated fat (red meat, butter, whole milk, and whole milk cheeses), substituting fish and chicken for red meat, and consuming more plant foods (fruits, vegetables, whole-grain products, and legumes). These simple dietary alterations can lower total caloric intake as well. Many Americans are consuming less red meat these days. Beef consumption has dropped, while our intake of poultry and fish—which are lower in fat—have increased.

What is the difference between saturated and unsaturated fats?

Saturated fats are usually hard at room temperature and are found primarily in animal products (meat, eggs, lard, butter, cream, whole milk, whole milk cheeses). Saturated fats are also present in solid vegetable fats and heavily hydrogenated vegetable fats such as shortenings and certain margarines. Two vegetable oils, coconut and palm oil, are also rich in saturated fats. Saturated fats tend to elevate blood cholesterol levels.

Fats and oils that are usually liquid at room temperature are abundant in plant seed oils—safflower, sunflower, corn, soybean, cottonseed, sesame, and rapeseed (canola). These are mainly polyunsaturated and can help lower blood cholesterol levels when substituted for saturated fat in the diet. Monounsaturated fats—abundant in olive, peanut, and canola oils—also can help reduce blood cholesterol levels when they replace saturated fats.

How important is dietary restriction of cholesterol?

Since cholesterol is manufactured in the body, dietary restriction may not have much effect on blood cholesterol levels. However, some individuals with elevated blood cholesterol levels may benefit from dietary restriction to 100–300 milligrams of cholesterol per day, which requires limiting one's intake of egg yolks (one to three per week) and organ meats. Egg substitutes contain no cholesterol but may contain an undesirable level of fat.

Is it a good idea to use "low cholesterol" products?

Don't be fooled by advertising hype! Heart disease prevention should begin with an assessment of *all* risk factors and be followed by changes to a healthier lifestyle. If you need to modify your diet, remember that lowering the fat content (especially the saturated fat content) is far more important than lowering the cholesterol content. Thus, dabbling with "low-cholesterol" products without addressing the important issues will do you little if any good.

Unfortunately, some manufacturers make "no cholesterol" claims even for products that are high in fat. Your best policy is to ignore the sales slogans and check the ingredients on the product label.

How does dietary fiber affect blood cholesterol level?

Soluble fiber—abundant in oat bran, oatmeal, dried beans and peas, and some fruits—can help lower total cholesterol and LDL levels. Corn bran, rice bran, carrots, and several citrus fruits may also help. But don't overdo it, because too much fiber can cause abdominal cramps and bloating. These problems can be minimized by increasing fiber content gradually over a period of weeks rather than suddenly.

I've heard that taking niacin supplements can lower blood cholesterol levels. Is that correct?

Yes, but *self-treatment* with niacin is unwise. The prevention and treatment of heart disease should be approached in a comprehensive manner. A preventive program should take all risk factors into account, not just blood cholesterol level. If someone's cholesterol level is high, attention should be paid to both exercise and diet. Normally, a cholesterol-lowering drug will not be prescribed unless it appears that dietary modification and exercise are unable to correct the problem. If a drug is appropriate, the choice and dosage of the drug will depend on factors that require medical training to evaluate properly.

In some individuals, high doses of niacin are very effective in lowering total cholesterol and LDL levels and raising the HDL level. But it also can damage the liver and elevate blood sugar and uric acid levels. For this reason, people who take niacin should have medical supervision with periodic blood tests to detect trouble before it becomes serious. Minor side effects (flushing and burning of the skin) are less common with sustained-release niacin than with regular (crystalline) niacin, but serious side effects are more common with the sustained-release variety.

In addition to single-ingredient niacin, most health food stores sell products composed of niacin, oat bran fiber, fish oils, lecithin, and/or various other ingredients. These formulations are neither rational nor safe for self-treatment.

Does sodium cause heart disease?

A diet high in sodium can contribute to the development of hypertension (high blood pressure), which is one of the risk factors for heart disease. In some patients, hypertension can be reduced with a low-sodium diet—but only in those who are "sodium-sensitive."

Twenty percent of the U.S. population has or will develop hypertension; one-third of these individuals are sodium-sensitive. The blood pressure of non-sensitive individuals does not increase with high sodium intakes. Since hypertension often produces no symptoms, blood pressure should be checked periodically.

Should everyone try to minimize dietary sodium?

Sodium is an essential mineral, important in the regulation of body fluids and other bodily functions. However, sodium restriction is essential for sodium-sensitive individuals. There is no laboratory test to determine sodium sensitivity. But when high blood pressure is diagnosed, the physician will usually suggest a trial of sodium reduction. A favorable response may avoid the need for medication.

Sodium is naturally present in most foods. Drinking water (especially softened water) also contains sodium. Salt is added to many processed foods as a preservative and for flavor, but the major dietary source of sodium is table salt. For moderate sodium restriction, you can eliminate the use of salt at the table and in cooking, and minimize your intake of the processed foods high in sodium:

• *Meats:* smoked, dried, cured, or salty items such as bacon, corned beef, hot dogs, luncheon meats, sausage, and canned fish

• *Other protein foods:* processed cheese, salted nuts, and peanut butter (with salt added)

• *Fruits and vegetables:* canned vegetables, certain frozen vegetables (peas, lima beans, mixed vegetables, and those packaged with seasonings or sauces), pickled beets, sauerkraut, tomato juice, and olives

• *Grain foods:* biscuits, crackers, pretzels, and snack foods (unless they are low-sodium)

• *Miscellaneous:* bouillon, condiments, soups and sauces, certain medications including antacids and aspirin.

Does use of a salt substitute actually decrease sodium intake?

Some salt substitutes consist of potassium chloride and sodium chloride, and contain about half the sodium of regular table salt. Research indicates that people who tend to use a large amount of regular salt will probably also use a large quantity of salt substitute. Substitutes made from sodium-free herbs and spices may be a preferable choice for those who are heavy-handed with the salt shaker. Sea salt contains as much sodium as table salt.

Many people habitually salt their food without tasting it first. Try tasting your food first before adding seasoning. You may find it isn't necessary to reach for the salt shaker after all.

Note: Don't use potassium or aluminum salt substitutes unless prescribed by your physician. For some individuals, unlimited intakes may be undesirable and excesses can prove toxic.

Does dietary calcium affect blood pressure?

Several studies have found an association between low-calcium diets and high blood pressure, indicating that calcium may exert some sort of protective effect. But don't start megadosing with calcium supplements! Simply include several daily servings from the Milk and Cheese Group, as recommended. If you are restricting sodium, avoid the saltier selections such as processed cheese.

Is it true that increasing potassium in the diet may help to decrease high blood pressure?

Some studies have shown that an increased dietary intake of potassium may reduce blood pressure in hypertensive patients, even if the diet is high in sodium. However, unless potassium depletion occurs with diuretics prescribed to lower the blood pressure, supplements are unnecessary because potassium is abundant in many foods. Potassium-rich foods include bananas, citrus and most other fruits, avocados, dried beans, potatoes, tomatoes, and leafy green vegetables.

Is sugar a culprit in heart disease?

No. In moderate amounts, sucrose (table sugar) has no known effect on the development of atherosclerosis or heart disease. However, if calories are consumed in excess and weight is gained, blood cholesterol levels usually increase. Overweight individuals also tend to have high blood pressure, another risk factor for heart disease. High-fat diets are more likely than high-carbohydrate diets to lead to obesity. Rich sweets—such as pies, cakes, cookies, and pastries—are often high in fat as well as calories.

What is the best advice for preventing heart disease?

To help prevent heart disease, you need to eliminate as many of the risk factors as you possibly can. So be sure to keep your weight under control, exercise regularly, and eat a well balanced diet. If your blood cholesterol is elevated, a diet low in saturated fat and cholesterol and high in soluble fiber may benefit your health. If your blood pressure is high, you may need to lose weight and moderate your sodium intake. And above all—don't smoke cigarettes.

Dietary modifications should be discussed with your physician, who may suggest consulting a dietitian or nutritionist for guidance in menu-planning. Cholesterol-lowering drugs should seldom be used unless these other measures fail to produce satisfactory results.

What is the Pritikin diet?

The Pritikin Program is promoted for prevention and treatment of a number of common diseases, including high blood pressure, heart disease, and diabetes. The program encourages vigorous physical activity and weight control and forbids cigarette smoking. The Pritikin diet emphasizes "complex" carbohydrates (cereal grains, legumes, potatoes, and other starchy foods), with fat intake limited to only 5 to 10 percent of total daily calories. This is so low in fat that few people are able to follow it on a long-term basis. The diet also is low in cholesterol and sodium, and it restricts the intake of refined carbohydrates (sugar, syrups, and highly processed grain foods such as white bread and polished rice). Coffee, tea, and alcohol are not allowed.

A few research teams have performed coronary artery studies (angiograms) on individuals with known heart disease who followed a diet with only 10 percent of total calories as fat. Many of these individuals achieved actual *regression* of their atherosclerosis. However, no published long-range study has compared the Pritikin diet to the less stringent diets (20 or 30 percent fat) advocated by the American Heart Association. Thus it is not clear whether dropping fat content to extremely low levels is worth the considerable effort required to do this.

How is cancer related to diet?

In 1982, the National Academy of Sciences (NAS) Committee on Diet, Nutrition, and Cancer issued what they called "interim dietary guidelines" in a thick report called *Diet, Nutrition and Cancer*. These guidelines were similar to the "Dietary Goals" of the 1970s and the U.S. Department of Agriculture's "Dietary Guidelines" that followed soon afterward. Like their predecessors, the "interim dietary guidelines" were greeted with controversy.

Although the NAS committee concluded that the data available were not sufficient to quantify the contribution of diet to the overall cancer risk or to determine the percent reduction in risk that might be achieved by dietary modification, they made public the following dietary suggestions:

• Reduce intake of fat, both saturated and unsaturated, from the current average of 40 percent to 30 percent of total calories.

• Include fruits, vegetables, and whole grains in the daily diet. Emphasize foods high in vitamin C and carotene, and the cruciferous vegetables (e.g., cauliflower, cabbage, broccoli, Brussels sprouts), but avoid high-dose vitamin supplements.

• Minimize intake of salt-cured, salt-pickled and smoked foods (such as bacon, bologna, hot dogs, smoked sausages, smoked fish, and ham).

• Drink alcohol only in moderation (especially if you smoke).

Although these interim guidelines were based on epidemiological data, animal studies, and experimental evidence from human studies, much of these data were (and still are) incomplete. The NAS committee also concluded that the following dietary components should be studied further:

• *Total caloric intake*. In animals, reduced food intake decreases the age-specific incidence of cancer.

- *Cholesterol.* The relationship of dietary intake and the incidence of cancer is unclear.
- *Protein.* Diets high in protein may be associated with certain cancers, but evidence is inconclusive because most diets high in protein are also high in fat.
- *Fiber.* If intake has any effect on certain cancers, it may be due to specific components of fiber.
- *Carbohydrates.* Any evidence of a role in carcinogenesis is unclear.
- *Selenium.* Studies suggest a protective role against cancer, but effects have been observed only in animals.
- *Other nutrients.* Insufficient data exist to determine the roles in carcinogenesis of vitamin E, iron, zinc, copper, molybdenum, arsenic, iodide, cadmium, and lead.

The NAS committee stated, "It is highly likely that the United States will eventually have the option of adopting a diet that reduces its incidence of cancer by approximately one-third." Yet they also concluded: "But it is not now, and may never be, possible to specify a diet that protects all people against all forms of cancer."

What are the major criticisms of the National Academy of Sciences diet-cancer report?

The report included an extensive literature survey and drew acclaim as well as criticism from food industry and health professionals. Its most serious drawback was probably the fact that most of its many reservations and uncertainties were not contained in the report's summary or in most of the news releases. As a result, there were significant discrepancies between the media reports and the report itself. Incomplete scientific research was oversimplified and sensationalized. Instead of waiting until solid evidence was available, educated speculations replaced documented evidence.

What do nutritionists now suggest?

First of all, try not to become obsessed with imaginary dangers lurking in your food. Needless worrying about unproven carcinogens won't improve your physical health and can damage your emotional health. Simply enjoy a variety of foods in moderate amounts from among and within the Basic Four Food Groups.

If dietary change is not the primary solution, how else can we protect ourselves against cancer?

You need to be able to separate the real risks from the hypothetical ones. And you should face the fact that the following risk factors for cancer are under your own control:

• *Cigarette smoking:* This is by far the most dangerous cancer-causing activity. So, if you don't smoke, don't start. If you do smoke, quit. (Information and advice about quitting are available from the American Cancer Society and the American Lung Association.) And if you find yourself inhaling other people's cigarette smoke, protest. It's *your* health that's at stake.

• *Alcoholic beverages:* Heavy drinkers run a greater risk of developing certain cancers than do nondrinkers. This risk is significantly greater in cigarette smokers.

• *Sunshine:* The sun's ultraviolet rays are a primary cause of skin cancer. So, if you spend much time in the sun, use a sunscreen with a high skin protection factor rating (SPF 15 or higher), especially if you are fair or have sensitive skin.

• *Sexual behavior and reproduction:* The evidence points to a connection between sexual behavior and reproduction and the incidence of certain cancers. For example, cervical cancer occurs more frequently in women who begin having sexual relations before age 17, and women who are childless after age 30 have an increased risk of breast cancer.

• *Occupational factors:* Long-term exposure to certain chemicals in the workplace can increase the risk for certain cancers. The potential risks need to be weighed against any known benefits. Meanwhile, handle all chemicals with care, and follow the directions and government regulations for use in order to at least minimize your own safety risks.

• *Medical radiation:* Most forms of radiation from x-rays can cause cancer. However, radiation is a valuable medical tool in the diagnosis and treatment of many diseases, including cancer. Doctors who recommend x-ray examinations believe that the potential benefits far outweigh the risks involved. Your best protection lies in selecting a doctor who uses good judgment.

• *Diet:* Overweight women are more likely to develop uterine cancer, and populations following a high-fat, low-fiber diet have higher rates of cancer of the breast, colon, and prostate. Insoluble fiber adds moisture and bulk to the stools and increases the rate at which food moves through the colon. This decreases intestinal "transit time," helping to prevent constipation and diverticulosis, an outpouching of the intestinal wall that can lead to diverticulitis (an inflammation). All diet-cancer links need more research, but the current scientific consensus is that a varied diet is the best course to follow.

Will eating certain vegetables diminish the carcinogenic effects of cigarette smoking?

Absolutely nothing you can put into your mouth will erase the dangers associated with placing a cigarette between your lips! The health hazards of cigarette smoking are well documented, and a warning appears on every cigarette pack sold in the U.S. today. Claims that nutritional supplements or special diets can lessen the carcinogenic effects of cigarette smoking should be regarded as misleading. The only true way to reduce the risk is to kick the smoking habit.

Some studies indicate that a diet rich in vegetable sources of carotenes, vitamins A, C, and E, and other factors may reduce the risk of certain cancers. This theory is still "green," but smokers could certainly do themselves and others a favor by popping carrot sticks instead of cigarettes into their mouth!

Are fiber pills worthwhile?

Adequate amounts of fiber can be obtained quite easily from food. Fiber supplements have several disadvantages: they may inhibit the absorption of certain minerals; they don't provide any nutrients; the long-term effects are unknown; and they add bulk to the food budget. In addition, use of fiber supplements can lead to a dependency on such pills to maintain "regularity."

What about other "anti-cancer" supplements?

Although the NAS report stated clearly that the use of supplements is *not* advisable, advertisements for anti-cancer nutrient-containing pills and potions appeared soon after the press publicized the committee's findings. These supplements were a direct—as well as an indirect—rip-off because the quantities of so-called protective factors (e.g., carotene) were too small to exert a significant effect on the body.

Since the ads were clearly fraudulent, the Federal Trade Commission was able to drive these products from the marketplace. But some supplement manufacturers still mention the NAS report and suggest that if you aren't eating foods rich in beta-carotene and other "protective" nutrients, supplementation might make sense. Others describe how various antioxidants are being studied to see whether supplements can help prevent cancer, but the results are not yet available. Most nutrition scientists doubt that people who eat properly can decrease their cancer risk by taking supplements.

Might a low-fat diet lead to the development of cancer?

Various studies have found an association between low cholesterol levels and certain cancers. However, it is not known whether the low cholesterol levels contributed to the development of the cancers or whether the presence of cancer caused the cholesterol levels to fall. Regardless, the proven cardiovascular benefit of maintaining a reasonable cholesterol level is far greater than any unproven risk of getting cancer.

Will a high-fat diet cause cancer?

Populations on low-fat diets tend to have a lower incidence of certain cancers—including colon and breast—than populations who consume large amounts of high-fat foods. Some scientists believe that it is an excess of *total* calories, not just fat-calories, that may contribute to the development of certain cancers. Others point to the overall reduction in consumption of fruits and vegetables that usually accompanies a diet high in fat. Still other researchers theorize that the presence of excess body weight—regardless of the source of the excess calories—is responsible for an increased cancer risk.

Since it is still too early to indict specific dietary components and to recommend others as definite factors in cancer prevention and cure, the moderate approach is most prudent. A diet in which fat comprises 30 percent or less of total calories is desirable anyway, as is an eating plan that includes generous servings of fruits, vegetables, and whole grains. Eat well, eat smart, exercise well, and don't smoke cigarettes. Increased health and vitality will be your reward.

APPENDIX A: RECOMMENDED DIETARY ALLOWANCES (1989)

These values, expressed as daily averages, are intended to provide for individual variations among normal persons as they live in the United States under usual environmental stresses. The heights and weights are medians for Americans in the listed ranges. The National Research Council recommends that diets be based on a variety of common foods in order to provide other nutrients for which human requirements are less well defined.

	Age (years)	Wt. (lbs)	Height (Inches)	Fat-Soluble Vitamins				C (mg)	Water-Soluble Vitamins					
				A[a] (µg RE)	D[b] (µg)	E (mg α-TE)[c]	K (µg)		Thiamin (mg)	Riboflavin (mg)	Niacin (mg)	B6 (µg)	Folate (µg)	B12 (µg)
Infants	0.0–0.5	13	24	375	7.5	3	5	30	0.3	0.4	5	0.3	25	0.3
	0.5–1.0	20	28	375	10	4	10	35	0.4	0.5	6	0.6	35	0.5
Children	1–3	29	35	400	10	6	15	40	0.7	0.8	9	1.0	50	0.7
	4–6	44	44	500	10	7	20	45	0.9	1.1	12	1.1	75	1.0
	7–10	62	52	700	10	7	30	45	1.0	1.2	13	1.4	100	1.4
Males	11–14	99	62	1,000	10	10	45	50	1.3	1.5	17	1.7	150	2.0
	15–18	145	69	1,000	10	10	65	60	1.5	1.8	20	2.0	200	2.0
	19–24	160	70	1,000	10	10	70	60	1.5	1.7	19	2.0	200	2.0
	25–50	174	70	1,000	5	10	80	60	1.5	1.7	19	2.0	200	2.0
	51+	170	68	1,000	5	10	80	60	1.2	1.4	15	2.0	200	2.0
Females	11–14	101	62	800	10	8	45	50	1.1	1.3	15	1.4	150	2.0
	15–18	120	64	800	10	8	55	60	1.1	1.3	15	1.5	180	2.0
	19–24	128	65	800	10	8	60	60	1.1	1.3	15	1.6	180	2.0
	25–50	138	64	800	5	8	65	60	1.1	1.3	15	1.6	180	2.0
	51+	143	63	800	5	8	65	60	1.0	1.2	13	1.6	180	2.0
Pregnant				800	10	10	65	70	1.5	1.6	17	2.2	400	2.2
Lactating, 1st 6 months				1,300	10	12	65	95	1.6	1.8	20	2.1	280	2.6
Lactating, 2nd 6 months				1,200	10	11	65	90	1.6	1.7	20	2.1	260	2.6

[a] 1 RE (retinol equivalent) = 1 µg retinol or 6 µg beta-carotene
[b] As cholecalciferol; 10 mg cholecalciferol = 400 International Units (IU) of vitamin D
[c] 1 mg α-TE = approximately 1 IU   1 µg = one millionth of a gram

1989 RECOMMENDED DIETARY ALLOWANCES (CONTINUED)

	Age (years)	Weight (lbs)	Height (inches)	Protein (grams)	Minerals						
					Calcium (mg)	Phosphorus (mg)	Magnesium (mg)	Iron (mg)	Zinc (mg)	Iodine (µg)	Selenium (µg)
Infants	0.0–0.5	13	24	13	400	300	40	6	5	40	10
	0.5–1.0	20	28	14	600	500	60	10	5	50	15
Children	1–3	29	35	16	800	800	80	10	10	70	20
	4–6	44	44	24	800	800	120	10	10	90	20
	7–10	62	52	28	800	800	170	10	10	120	30
Males	11–14	99	62	45	1,200	1,200	270	12	15	150	40
	15–18	145	69	59	1,200	1,200	400	12	15	150	50
	19–24	160	70	58	1,200	1,200	350	10	15	150	70
	25–50	174	70	63	800	800	350	10	15	150	70
	51+	170	68	63	800	800	350	10	15	150	70
Females	11–14	101	62	46	1,200	1,200	280	15	12	150	45
	15–18	120	64	44	1,200	1,200	300	15	12	150	50
	19–24	128	65	46	1,200	1,200	280	15	12	150	55
	25–50	138	64	50	800	800	280	15	12	150	55
	51+	143	63	50	800	800	280	10	12	150	55
Pregnant				60	1,200	1,200	320	30	15	175	65
Lactating, 1st 6 months				65	1,200	1,200	355	15	19	200	75
Lactating, 2nd 6 months				62	1,200	1,200	340	15	16	200	75

Appendix B

Glossary

Acidosis: The condition in which body fluids are excessively acidic from an accumulation of acids, due to diabetes, fasting, low-carbohydrate intake, diarrhea, vomiting, dehydration, kidney disease, or other conditions.

Acupuncture: A treatment method based on the belief that inserting needles into various body areas can heal the body by balancing its "life forces."

Additives: Chemical compounds added to foods to improve flavor, appearance, shelf life, and/or nutritive value.

Aflatoxins: Poisonous substances found in moldy peanuts, wheat, corn, rice, and other products. Aflatoxins can cause cancer in animals.

Amino acids: Some twenty-two basic chemical compounds that are the building blocks of proteins. The eight that cannot be made by the body are called "essential" and must be obtained from food.

Anemia: A group of disorders characterized by deficient oxygen-carrying capacity of the blood caused by a defect in the number and/or quality of the red blood cells.

Anorexia nervosa: A psychological disorder resulting in self-starvation to the point of emaciation, malnutrition, and sometimes death. Most victims are adolescent girls and young women.

Antioxidant: Any substance that inhibits chemical reactions promoted by oxygen. Antioxidants can thus act as preservatives. Common antioxidants include vitamin C, vitamin E, BHA (butylated hydroxyanisole), and BHT (butylated hydroxytoluene).

Arteriosclerosis: A disease characterized by thickening and hardening of artery walls, which cause the arteries to become narrower and less elastic.

Aspartame: A low-calorie sugar substitute composed mainly of two amino acids (aspartic acid and phenylalanine) naturally present in food. It is about two hundred times as sweet as sugar.

Atherosclerosis: A type of arteriosclerosis characterized by cholesterol-filled fatty deposits that develop inside artery walls.

Balanced diet: A diet composed of a variety of foods from among and within the Basic Four Food Groups. Balanced diets provide the required nutrients in adequate amounts.

Basic Four: A term for the classification of foods into groups on the basis of their main nutrients. The four basic groups are: Fruit and Vegetable Group, Cereal and Grain Group, Milk and Cheese Group, and Meat and Alternates Group. A balanced diet can be obtained by eating appropriate amounts of a variety of foods from each group daily.

Beriberi: A deficiency disease caused by inadequate intake of thiamin and characterized by loss of appetite, gastrointestinal disturbances, nervous system disorders, and heart irregularities.

Biochemistry: The science of the intricate chemical processes that govern life for plants and animals, including humans.

Bran: The coarse outer layer of grains that supply dietary fiber, most of which is indigestible.

Caffeine: A potentially addictive cardiac and central nervous system stimulant found in varying amounts in coffee, tea, cocoa, cola beverages, and certain medications.

Calorie: A unit of measure that expresses the energy value of foods. Physicists use the word to mean the amount of energy needed to raise one gram of water one degree Celsius. When nutrition scientists refer to the number of calories in food, they use the unit "kilocalorie" or "Calorie" (spelled with a capital C), which is actually 1,000 small calories. In common usage, however, the term "calorie," although spelled with a small c, means kilocalorie. Fat yields 9 calories per gram, while protein and carbohydrate each yield 4 calories per gram. Alcohol yields 7 calories per gram.

Cancer: A term encompassing a large group of diseases characterized by unregulated cell growth.

Carbohydrate: Chemically neutral compounds (starches, sugars, and celluloses) composed of carbon, hydrogen, and oxygen. Starches and sugars are a ready source of food energy.

Carcinogen: A cancer-causing substance.

Caries: Tooth decay.

Cariogenic substance: Any substance that favors the development of tooth decay.

Carotenes: A group of yellow pigments found in various plant and animal tissues. Beta-carotene is the precursor of vitamin A. Carotenes are abundant in yellow vegetables such as carrots and squash. An excessive intake of carotenes can cause yellowed skin.

Cellulite: A fanciful nonmedical term for the wrinkled fat found mainly in the thigh/buttocks area.

Cellulose: The principal fiber of bran (also found in fruits and vegetables), which can be present with hemicellulose and lignin to form the supporting structure for plants.

Chemical: Any substance made up of the elements that compose all matter, including food and human beings.

Chiropractic: A system of health care based on the false theory that most ailments are the result of misaligned spinal bones. Chiropractors are not licensed to perform surgery or prescribe drugs, but many of them advocate the use of food supplements that are unnecessary and/or irrational.

Cholesterol: A waxy, fat-like substance essential to life and present in every animal cell. Cholesterol is manufactured by several body tissues (particularly the liver). It is found only in foods of animal origin. Egg yolk and organ meats are especially high in cholesterol, while fatty meats, shrimp, butter, cream, whole milk, and whole milk cheeses contain significant amounts.

"Clinical ecology": A pseudoscience based on the belief that multiple symptoms are triggered by hypersensitivity to common foods and chemicals.

Colitis: A group of conditions characterized by inflammation of the large intestine (colon).

Controlled experiment: An experiment in which the results of doing something are compared to the results of doing something else to similar groups of people. For example, people treated with a medicine may be compared to similar people receiving an inert substance (placebo).

Coronary: A term referring to the arteries that supply blood to the heart.

Cyclamate: A non-nutritive sugar substitute. Cyclamate is presently banned in the United States because of suspicions of carcinogenicity, but it is used in Canada and many other countries.

Desirable Weight: Formerly called "ideal weight," it is the weight at which most people will live longest—determined by insurance actuarial data to be the average weight at age 25 for males and females for each specific height.

Diabetes: A disease characterized by the inability to make enough insulin to metabolize carbohydrates. The most common form, which occurs in later life, can usually be controlled by maintaining proper weight and diet.

Diathermy: The use of high-frequency currents to heat body areas and temporarily increase blood flow to these areas.

Dietitian: Registered Dietitians (R.D.s) are nutrition professionals, usually bachelor- or master-level graduates, who have additional clinical experience, have passed a comprehensive written examination, and participate regularly in continuing education programs approved by the American Dietetic Association.

Digestion: The process by which food is broken down by the gastrointestinal system into absorbable nutrients.

Diuretic: A drug (or food substance) that induces loss of body fluids by increasing the secretion of urine.

Double-blind test: An experiment in which neither the experimental subjects nor those responsible for the treatment or data collection know which subjects receive the treatment being tested and which receive something else (such as a placebo).

Emulsifier: A product that keeps fat particles suspended in another substance. Emulsifiers are commonly used in fat-containing food products such as salad dressings, ice cream, and packaged mixes. Egg yolk and soybeans contain the emulsifier lecithin.

Energy: Food energy is the caloric content of foods.

Enrichment: The addition of nutrients to foods to return their nutrient value approximately to the levels present before processing.

Enzymes: Protein substances that trigger and speed up chemical changes within the body.

Epidemiology: The science that studies the relationships between environment (including diet) and diseases in population groups. Epidemiologists seek to explain the differences in the incidence of diseases among population groups.

Essential nutrients: Specific nutrients that cannot be synthesized by the body and must therefore be obtained from foods.

Exchange lists: Food groupings developed by the American Diabetes Association and the American Dietetic Association. Foods are classified according to similarities in caloric and nutrient values for interchangeable use in menu planning for diabetics and others on special diets.

Faddist: In nutrition, one who attributes nonexistent health-promoting properties to foods or food substances.

"Fast food": Restaurant items that are prepared and served quickly and usually can be eaten out of one's hand. More appropriately called "fast-service foods," some common examples are hamburgers, pizza, doughnuts, fried chicken, and fried fish.

Fat: A chemical compound of three fatty acids connected to glycerol. Fats may be animal or vegetable in origin and are solid or liquid at room temperature.

Fatty acids: Components of fat that can be classified as "saturated" or "unsaturated." Linoleic acid, which is essential, is unsaturated.

Fiber: Plant material consisting mostly of indigestible carbohydrates. "Dietary fiber" includes at least five different components: cellulose, hemicellulose, lignin, pectin, and gum. "Crude fiber" is what remains after laboratory breakdown of food with acid and alkali.

Fluoridation: A valuable public health procedure by which the concentration of the mineral nutrient fluoride in water supplies is adjusted to about one part fluoride to one million parts water (1 ppm). Use of fluoridated water throughout childhood greatly reduces the incidence of tooth decay.

Food combining: Dietary practice based on the incorrect notion that certain food combinations can cause or correct ill health.

Food irradiation: Application of ionizing radiation (x-rays or beta rays) to foods to kill organisms, inhibit sprouting, or delay ripening.

Food supplement: Product used to provide nutrients in addition to those found in one's diet.

Fortification: Addition of nutrient(s) to a food to increase the nutrient value above that available naturally.

Fructose: A simple sugar that comprises half of the compound sucrose (table sugar) and is the predominant sugar in some fruits.

Galactose: A simple sugar that, with glucose, forms lactose (milk sugar).

Gastrointestinal ("G.I."): Pertaining to the digestive tract.

Glucose: A simple sugar that is the body's basic fuel. It is also called dextrose.

Glycogen: The body's chief storage form of carbohydrate. Small amounts, stored in the liver and muscles, are released as needed for conversion to glucose.

Goiter: Enlargement of the thyroid gland.

Gout: A disease in which uric acid accumulates in the blood and can form painful deposits in the joints, particularly of the toes.

Gums: The resin-like indigestible substances found in plants.

GRAS: The abbreviation for "Generally Recognized as Safe."

HDL (high-density lipoproteins): Lipoproteins that transport cholesterol to the liver to be disposed of. A high proportion of HDL in the blood may indicate a low risk for coronary heart disease. HDL is sometimes referred to as "good cholesterol."

"Health food": A misleading term which has no legal definition but suggests that a food has a unique or special health-promoting quality.

"Holistic" medicine: Treatment of the whole person. Although this philosophy is part of traditional medicine, many practitioners who call themselves "holistic" suggest that they have something special to offer. Such practitioners often advocate the use of unnecessary food supplements and other questionable "health" practices.

Homeopathy: A system of treatment based on the false theory that infinitesimal dosages of various substances can be potent remedies.

Hormone: A protein that is produced by a body organ or gland and travels through the bloodstream to other body areas to stimulate function.

Hydrogenation: A controllable chemical process used to convert unsaturated fats from liquid to semisolid form by the addition of hydrogen to the fat. This lengthens shelf life of the product and improves physical properties such as spreadability. Hydrogenation is used to make margarine from vegetable oils.

Hyperactivity (hyperkinesis): Excessive activity due to many different psychological and perhaps physiological causes.

Hyperalimentation: A method of intravenous feeding that provides the essential nutrients and calories needed to sustain life for long periods of time. This method is usually used for very ill individuals who are unable to eat for physiological or psychological reasons.

Hypercholesterolemia: An excess of cholesterol in the blood. (Occasionally referred to as hypercholesteremia.)

Hypertension: A condition in which blood pressure is higher than normal. If resting blood pressure is above 140/90, diet and/or drug treatment may be prescribed.

Hypoglycemia: A rare illness in which blood sugar drops very low. Also, a common "fad" diagnosis.

Insulin: Pancreatic hormone important in the regulation of blood sugar. Inadequate secretion causes diabetes, and treatment includes proper diet with or without insulin injections or other drug therapy.

Iridology: System of medical diagnosis based on the absurd theory that ill health in every bodily part is reflected in the iris of the eye. Practitioners of iridology usually advocate the use of unnecessary nutritional supplements and other questionable "health" practices.

"Junk food": A misleading term used to suggest that snack items, fast foods, and processed foodstuffs lack nutritional value. Any food can be "junk" if eaten in such excess that it unbalances one's diet.

Lactation: The period of secreting milk for breast-feeding purposes.

Lactose: A disaccharide composed of glucose and galactose. Lactose is found only in milk and foods made with milk, and it is added to some processed foods. Many individuals are unable to tolerate large amounts of lactose because they lack the enzyme lactase. But most of these people are able to ingest small quantities without gastrointestinal upset.

Laetrile: An ineffective cancer "remedy" derived from apricot pits. It is sometimes called "vitamin B_{17}," although it is not a vitamin.

LDL (low-density lipoproteins): Lipoproteins that may transport cholesterol to storage sites throughout the body. A high proportion of LDL in the blood may indicate increased risk for developing coronary heart disease. LDL is sometimes referred to as "bad cholesterol."

Lecithin: A phospholipid made in the liver and present in most foods of animal origin. Commercial lecithin comes from egg yolks or soybeans.

Legumes: A group of vegetables that includes peas and beans, including black beans, black-eyed peas, broad beans, chick peas, kidney beans, lima beans, pinto beans, soybeans, lentils, split peas, and peanuts.

Lignin: A noncarbohydrate fiber that helps form plant structure and is present in grains (especially rye and wheat), vegetables, fruits, and nuts.

Linoleic acid: The unsaturated fatty acid essential for humans and present in many vegetable oils such as sunflower, safflower, corn, and soy oil.

Lipid: A general term for fat and other substances with chemical and physical properties similar to those of fat.

Lipoproteins: Fat-protein combinations that transport fats and proteins in the blood and are classified according to density.

Macrobiotic: A word meaning "long life." The macrobiotic diet is a primarily vegetarian diet that includes small amounts of fish, but excludes meat, poultry, dairy products, certain fruits, coffee, and most processed foods.

Maltose: A disaccharide, composed of two glucose units, that is found in malt products and sprouting seeds.

Megadose: A dose that is much higher (often ten times higher) than the Recommended Dietary Allowance. Megadoses of most nutrients can have toxic effects.

Megaloblastic anemia: A serious condition in which the red blood cells are immature and abnormally large due to deficiency or malabsorption of folic acid or vitamin B_{12}; symptoms include weakness, numbness, gastrointestinal upset, nerve damage, and heart failure. Strict vegetarians are susceptible unless they eat vitamin B_{12}-fortified foods or take a B_{12} supplement.

Metabolism: A term used to describe the chemical processes that occur in the body.

Minerals: Naturally occurring inorganic elements. Those known to be essential to humans include sodium, potassium, calcium, phosphorus, iron, iodide, copper, cobalt, magnesium, chloride, chromium, manganese, fluoride, sulfur, selenium, zinc, and molybdenum.

Monounsaturated fats: Liquid at room temperature, these fats can lower blood cholesterol levels when they replace a substantial amount of saturated fat in the diet. They are abundant in olive, canola, and peanut oil.

"Natural": A misleading term used to suggest that a product is safer and more nutritious.

Naturopathy: A system of health care which advocates light, heat, air, water, and massage in place of conventional medical treatment. Naturopaths disfavor the use of drugs, but many advocate herbal extracts, unnecessary nutritional supplements, and other questionable "health" practices.

Nucleic acids: Substances found in cell nuclei. The most important nucleic acids, DNA and RNA, are part of the cell's reproductive apparatus.

Nutrients: Some fifty known food substances—including protein, fat, carbohydrate, vitamins, minerals, and water—that are required to nourish the body.

Nutrition: The science of foods, their components, and their relationship to health and disease.

Nutritionist: An expert in nutrition and/or dietetics. As used in this book, the term encompasses dietitians as well as others with accredited credentials in nutrition. A few states have laws that define the practice of nutrition and restrict use of the word "nutritionist" to qualified professionals. In most states, however, anyone can utilize this title whether qualified or not.

Obesity: Excessive body weight due to the presence of surplus fat.

Obesity is defined as 20 percent or more above desirable weight.

Omnivorous: Eating foods of both animal and vegetable origin.

"Organic" or *"Organically grown":* Misleading labels used by those who wish to suggest that foods grown without pesticides or chemical fertilizers are safer and/or more nutritious than conventionally grown foods.

Osteomalacia: A disease in which the bones become increasingly soft. Actually the adult form of rickets, the condition is due to deficiency in vitamin D and/or calcium.

Osteoporosis: A disease commonly affecting the elderly (primarily women) in which the bones become increasingly porous and brittle. Contributing factors may include inadequate intake of calcium, fluoride, vitamin D, and other nutrients, lack of exercise, and other lifestyle factors.

Overfat: Having excess body fat. Most overfat individuals are overweight, but some are not.

Overweight: Weighing between 10 and 20 percent more than the amount listed in a standard height-weight table.

Pectin: The principal fiber of apples, citrus fruits, and other fruits.

Pellagra: A deficiency disease caused by inadequate intake of niacin and characterized by dermatitis, diarrhea, dementia, and eventually death.

Pesticides: Chemicals used to control the pests and weeds that destroy plants grown for food and other purposes.

Phospholipid: A fatty substance containing a phosphate in place of one of the fatty acids. An example is lecithin.

Physiology: The science of the various chemical and physical functions of organisms, including humans.

Plaque: An arterial plaque is a fatty deposit in the wall of a blood vessel. Dental plaque is the bacterial film on the surface of the teeth.

Polyunsaturated fats: Fats that have room for several hydrogen atoms. These fats abound in plant seed oils (safflower, sunflower, cottonseed, canola, soybean, sesame, and walnut) and are liquid at room temperature. They are effective in lowering blood cholesterol when used to replace some of the saturated fat in the diet.

Postmenopausal: After the menopause, the period of life in which women undergo major hormonal changes and are no longer able to bear children.

Preservative: Any substance added to food to delay breakdown, prevent spoilage, and prolong shelf life. Common examples include salt, vitamin C, and vitamin E.

Precursor: A substance from which another substance is derived, commonly used to describe an inactive substance that is converted into an active enzyme, vitamin or hormone. Beta-carotene, for example, is a precursor of vitamin A.

Proteins: Compounds of amino acids, essential to tissue synthesis and the regulation of certain body functions.

Pseudonutritionist: One who claims to be a nutritionist but has no acceptable educational background or professional training. Usually such individuals promote questionable dietary advice and unnecessary nutritional supplements.

Quack: A pretender to knowledge. A nutrition quack is one who pretends to be knowledgeable about diet and health.

Quackery: The promotion of health fads by those who falsely pretend to be knowledgeable about medicine, typically regarding diet and health.

RDAs (Recommended Dietary Allowances): The levels of average daily intake for protein, eleven vitamins, and seven minerals considered to be adequate for healthy persons and used as a guide for evaluating the diets of population groups. The RDAs were first issued in 1943 by the Food and Nutrition Board of the Research Council (NRC) and have been revised periodically. The latest revision was published in 1989. Recently, the Food and Nutrition Board was made part of NRC's Institute of Medicine.

Reflexology: A pseudoscience based on the false theory that ill health is treatable by manipulation of body parts, primarily the hand or foot.

Rickets: A disease in children that results in abnormal bone formation, caused primarily by vitamin D deficiency and/or inadequate calcium.

Risk factor: A factor believed to contribute to the development of a disease. (For example, smoking, obesity, and high blood pressure are risk factors for heart disease.) A noncausative factor (such as a laboratory test) that accompanies or presages a disease is called a "marker."

Saturated fats: Fats in which the chains of carbon atoms are filled to capacity with hydrogen. These fats are found primarily in animal products (meat, eggs, lard, butter, cream, whole milk, and whole milk cheese) and are usually solid at room temperature. They are also found in liquid form in coconut and palm oils.

Scurvy: A deficiency disease caused by inadequate intake of vitamin C, characterized by bleeding gums, loss of teeth, poor wound healing, general pain, and fatigue.

Sodium: A mineral, found in most foods, that comprises 40 percent of table salt.

Starches: The digestible polysaccharides that, with the indigestible fibers, are referred to as complex carbohydrates.

Sterol: An alcohol of high molecular weight found in both animals and plants. Examples are cholesterol in animals and sitosterol in plants.

Sucrose: A sugar obtained from sugar cane or sugar beets and commonly known as table sugar (white granulated sugar). It is composed of a molecule of glucose and one of fructose. Sucrose is also found in some fruits.

Sugars: Simple carbohydrates, either mono- or disaccharides.

Synthetic: Term applied to compounds that are manufactured as opposed to those that are made naturally by living cells.

Tannins: Substances obtained from coffee, tea, cocoa, and certain other plants that are astringent in taste and toxic in high doses.

Thyroid: A gland in the neck that secretes hormones important in body metabolism. An iodide deficiency causes the gland to swell, a condition known as goiter.

Toxic: Poisonous.

Triglycerides: The primary form of fats (lipids) in the diet and the blood, and the usual storage form of fats in the body. Most triglycerides are synthesized in the body from glucose and fatty acids,

Turbinado sugar: So-called "raw" sugar, this brown form of sucrose is actually partially refined to remove impurities and is nutritionally similar to white sugar.

Unsaturated fats: Fats that contain less hydrogen than saturated fats. They are liquid or semisolid at room temperature.

Vitamins: Organic substances essential in small amounts for life and growth. Vitamins are commonly divided into two groups, based on solubility. The fat-soluble ones are A, D, E, and K. The water-soluble ones are C and the eight B-complex vitamins.

Appendix C

Recommended Reading

The following publications can help you to deepen and keep current your knowledge of nutrition. Most of the books can be obtained from bookstores, either directly or by special order. For items not usually available through bookstores, we have provided the publisher's address.

General nutrition

Aronson, V. *Thirty Days to Better Nutrition,* Prentice-Hall, 1987.

Baker, S. and Henry, R. *Parents' Guide to Nutrition,* Addison-Wesley, 1987.

Connor, S. and Connor, W. *The New American Diet,* Simon and Schuster, 1986.

Eisenberg, H. et al. *What to Eat When You're Expecting,* Workman, 1986.

Franz, M. et al. *Opening the Door to Good Nutrition,* International Diabetes Center (4959 Excelsior Boulevard, Minneapolis, MN 55416), 1985.

Franz, M. *Fast Food Facts,* International Diabetes Center (4959 Excelsior Blvd., Minneapolis, MN 55416), 1987.

Guthrie, H. *Introductory Nutrition, 7th edition,* Times Mirror Mosby, 1989.

Hamilton, E., Whitney, E., and Sizer, F. *Nutrition—Concepts and Controversies, 4th Edition,* West Publishing, 1988.

Herbert, V., and Subak-Sharpe, G., eds. *The Mount Sinai School of Medicine Complete Book of Nutrition.* St. Martin's Press, 1990.

Long, P. *The Nutritional Ages of Women—A Lifetime Guide to Eating Right for Health, Beauty, and Well-being,* Macmillan, 1986.

Recommended Dietary Allowances, 10th edition, National Research Council, Washington, D.C., 1989.

Stare, F. and Aronson, V. *Food for Fitness After Fifty,* J.B. Lippincott Co., 1987.

———. *Food for Today's Teens,* J. B. Lippincott Co., 1985.

Stare, F., Olson, R., and Whelan, E. *Balanced Nutrition—Beyond the Cholesterol Scare,* Bob Adams, Inc., Holbrook, MA, 1989.

Stern, B. *The Food Book—The Complete Guide to the Most Popular Brand Name Foods in the U.S.,* Dell, 1987.

U.S. Department of Agriculture. *Nutrition and Your Health—Dietary Guidelines for Americans, 3rd edition,* U.S. Government Printing Office (Superintendent of Documents, Washington, DC 20402), 1990.

U.S. Department of Agriculture. *Nutritive Value of Foods,* U.S. Government Printing Office (Superintendent of Documents, Washington, DC 20402), 1985.

U.S. Surgeon General. *U.S. Surgeon General's Report on Nutrition and Health,* U.S. Government Printing Office (Superintendent of Documents, Washington, DC 20402), 1988.

Food faddism and quackery

Barrett, S. *The Health Robbers—How to Protect Your Money and Your Life,* George F. Stickley Co., 1980.

Barrett, S. et al. *Health Schemes, Scams, and Frauds.* Consumer Reports Books, 1990.

Fried, J. *Vitamin Politics,* Prometheus Books, 1984.

Herbert, V. and Barrett, S. *Vitamins and "Health" Foods: The Great American Hustle,* J.B. Lippincott Co., 1981.

Marshall, C. *Vitamins & Minerals: Help or Harm?,* J.B. Lippincott Co., 1985.

Tyler, V. *The New Honest Herbal,* J.B. Lippincott Co., 1987.

Whelan, E. and Stare, F. *The 100% Natural, Purely Organic, Cholesterol-Free, Megavitamin, Low-Carbohydrate Nutrition Hoax,* Atheneum, 1983.

Yetiv, J. *Popular Nutritional Practices: A Scientific Appraisal,* Popular Medicine Press, 1986.

Weight control

Bennion, L. et al. *Straight Talk About Weight Control.*Consumer Reports Books, 1990.

California Dietetic Association. *Popular Diets—How They Rate,* Los Angeles District Dietetic Association, 1987.

Chernin, K. *The Hungry Self,* Harper and Row, 1985.

Ikeda, J. *Winning Weight Loss for Teens,* Bull Publishing Co., 1987.

Jonas, S. and Aronson, V. *The I Don't Eat (But I Can't Lose) Weight Loss Program,* Rawson Associates, 1989.

Lansky, V. *Fat-Proofing Your Children . . . So That They Never Become Diet-Addicted Adults,* Bantam, 1988.

Satter, E. *How to Get Your Kid to Eat . . . But Not Too Much,* Bull Publishing Co., 1987.

Stare, F. and Whelan, E. *The Harvard Square Diet,* Prometheus Books, 1987.

Stuart, R. and Jacobson, B. *Weight, Sex, and Marriage: A Delicate Balance,* W.W. Norton, 1987.

Exercise and sports nutrition

Addleman, F. *The Winning Edge—Nutrition for Athletic Fitness and Performance,* Prentice-Hall, 1984.

Cooper, K. and Cooper M. *The New Aerobics for Women,* Bantam, 1988.

Nieman, D. *The Sports Medicine Fitness Course,* Bull Publishing Co., 1986.

Shangold, M. *The Complete Sports Medicine Book for Women,* Simon and Schuster, 1985.

Turock, A. *Getting Physical—How to Stick with Your Exercise Program,* Doubleday, 1988.

Wilmore, J. *Sensible Fitness,* Leisure Press, 1986.

Cookbooks

American Diabetes Association. *American Diabetes Association Family Cookbook,* Prentice-Hall, 1984.

American Dietetic Association. *Dietitians' Food Favorites.* ADA (216 West Jackson Boulevard, Chicago, IL 60606), 1986.

American Heart Association. *American Heart Association Cookbook,* Ballantine, 1986.

Fletcher, A. *Eat Fish, Live Better,* Harper and Row, 1989.

Metropolitan Life Insurance Co. *Eat Well, Be Well Cookbook,* Simon and Schuster, 1986.

Robertson, L., Flinders, C., and Godfrey, B. *The New Laurel's Kitchen,* Ten Speed Press, 1986.

Roth, H. *Deliciously Simple,* New American Library, 1986.

Underwood, G. *Gourmet Light,* The Globe Pequot Press, 1985.

_____. *The Enlightened Gourmet,* The Globe Pequot Press, 1987.

Magazines and Newsletters

American Health, Box 3016, Harlan, IA 51593.

Consumer Reports, P.O. Box 53029, Boulder, CO 80322.

Consumer Reports Health Letter, P.O. Box 52148, Boulder, CO 80321.

Environmental Nutrition, 2112 Broadway, Suite 200, New York, NY 10023.

FDA Consumer, Superintendent of Documents, U.S. Government Printing Office, Washington, DC 20402.

Food News for Consumers, Superintendent of Documents, U.S. Government Printing Office, Washington, DC 20402.

Harvard Health Letter, P.O. Box 420300, Palm Coast, FL 32142.

Harvard Heart Letter, P.O. Box 420234, Palm Coast, FL 32142.

In Health, P.O. Box 56863, Boulder, CO 80322.

Mirkin Report, P.O. Box 6608, Silver Spring, MD 20916.

Nutrition Forum, P.O. Box 1747, Allentown, PA 18105.

Nutrition Today, Williams & Wilkins, 428 E. Preston Street, Baltimore, MD 21202.

Obesity and Health, Healthy Living Institute, Route 2, Box 905, Hettinger, ND 58639.

Priorities, American Council on Science and Health, 1995 Broadway, New York, NY 10023.

Running and FitNews, American Running and Fitness Association, 9310 Old Georgetown Road, Bethesda, MD 20814.

Sports-Medicine News, P.O. Box 986, Evanston, IL 60204.

Tufts University Diet and Nutrition Letter, P.O. Box 10948, Des Moines, IA 50940.

University of California, Berkeley Wellness Letter, P.O. Box 10922, Des Moines, IA 50940.

Index

"t" following a page number indicates a table.

Accreditation system, 40
Acerola berries, vitamin C from, 52
Acesulfame-K, 103
Acidophilus, 61-62
Acidosis, 187
Activated charcoal, 62
Acupuncture, 187
Acyclovir, 77
Additive(s)
    approval by FDA, 97-98
    beneficial effects, 95, 96-97
    cancer risk, 101-103, 104, 106-107
    definition, 95, 187
    Delaney Clause and, 102
    fear of, 96, 97, 109
    GRAS list, 98
    and hyperactivity, 105-106
    natural sources, 95
    need for, 96-97
    safety, 97-99
    truth about, 95-109

Advice, sources, 37-45, 198-201
Aflatoxins, 101, 187
Agriculture Department, U.S., 41
AIDS, 44, 83
Air Force Diet, 128t
Airola, Paavo, 71-72
Alcohol abuse complications, 157-158
Alcoholic beverages
    alcohol content, 154-156, 156t
    calorie content, 154-156, 156t
    and cancer, 158
    and heart disease, 159
    and malnutrition, 157,158
    and pregnancy, 159-160
Alfalfa, 62
Alfalfa tea, 62
Aloe vera, 62-63
"Alternative" health care, 29
American Academy of Allergy and Immunology, 33, 83
American Academy of Environmental Medicine, 40

American Academy of Pediatrics, 21, 54
American Association of Nutritional Consultants, 40
American College of Advancement in Medicine, 40
American College of Health Science, 126
American Council on Science and Health, 41, 44, 102
American Dental Association, 54
American Diabetes Association, 144
American Dietetic Association (ADA), 38, 41
American Holistic Medical Association, 40
American Institute of Nutrition, 39, 41
American Medical Association Department of Personal Health, 41
American Natural Hygiene Society, 40
American Nutritional Consultants Association, 41
American Nutritional Medical Association, 41
American Nutritionists Association, 41
American Quack Association, 41
American Society for Clinical Nutrition, 39, 41
Amino acids, 3t, 7-8, 63, 77, 187
  for athletes, 170
  in diet aids, 122-123
Amphetamines, 120
Amway Corporation, 26
Amygdalin, 76
Anemia, 187
  iron-deficiency, 21
  megaloblastic, 194
Annapolis Diet, 128t
Anorexia nervosa, 161, 164-166, 187
Antioxidants, 81, 187-188
Applied kinesiology, 31

Arteriosclerosis, 188
Asai, Kazuhiko, 70
Aspartame, 103-104, 188
Atherosclerosis, 172, 188
Atkins Diet, 128t
Aversive conditioning, 123

Balanced diet, 1, 188; *see also* Basic Four Food Groups
Barrett, Dr. Stephen, 27
Basic Four Food Groups, 5, 17-18, 18t, 20, 24, 25, 48, 49, 67, 87, 114, 147, 163, 170, 181, 188
  charts, and use of, 18t-19t
  and vegetarian diets, 134
Bee pollen, 63
Behavior modification, for weight control, 115-116
Benzocaine, 121
Beriberi, 25, 188
Bernadean University, 39
Beta-carotene, 50, 51-52
Beverly Hills Diet, 128t
BHA, 106-107
BHT, 106-107
Bile, 7
Bio-Diet, 128t
Biochemistry, 188
Bioflavonoids, 61, 64
Blackstrap molasses, 64
Blood pressure
  and calcium, 178
  and potassium, 178
  and sodium, 14
  among vegetarians, 140
Bloomingdale's Eat Healthy Diet, 128t
Bone meal, 44, 58-59, 64
Boron, 58
Bottled water, 160-161
Bovine somatotropin (BST), 161
Bran, 64-65, 188
Breakfast
  in "fast food" restaurant, 91
  importance of, 91, 163

Breakfast cereals, fortified, 55
Breastfeeding, nutritional
    advantages of, 21
Brewer's yeast, 65
Brown sugar, 148-149
Bruch, Hilde, 165
BST (bovine somatotropin), 161
Bulimia, 165, 166
Butylated hydroxyanisole; *see* BHA
Butylated hydroxytoluene; *see* BHT

Caffeine, 188
    adverse effects, 152-153
    and athletic performance, 152
    metabolism, 151
    sources, 150, 151, 153-154,
        154*t*, 168
    stimulant effects, 151, 152
Cal-Ban 3000, 122
Calcium, 13-14, 55, 59
    and blood pressure, 178
    deficiency, 13
    functions, 13
    and osteoporosis, 55
    for postmenopausal women, 55
    sources, 14, 67, 136*t*
Calories, 113, 188
    in alcoholic beverages, 22, 24,
        156*t*
    in body fat, 113-114, 115
    excess, as problem in U.S., 87
    nutrients and, 22
    sources of, 114
Calories Don't Count Diet, 128*t*
Cancer Control Society, 41
Cancer
    alcohol and, 158
    and blood cholesterol levels, 184
    and diet, 63, 180-184
    risk factors, 182-183
    selenium and, 58
    stomach, and BHA and BHT,
        106-107
    vitamin A and, 50-51
    vitamin C and, 52
"Candidiasis hypersensitivity," 83

Carbohydrate loading, 169
Carbohydrates, 8, 22, 188
    "complex," 9
    composition of, 2
Cardiomyopathy, 159
Carob, 65, 84
Carotenemia, 51
Carotenes, 51, 189
"Cellulite," 124-125, 189
Cellulose, 8, 189
Cereals, breakfast
    fortified, 55
    presweetened, 148
Charcoal, activated, 62
Chelated minerals, 64-65
Chelation therapy, 32
Chemical elements, essential, 2-3, 3*t*
Chinese Restaurant Syndrome, 107,
    108
Chiropractors, 34, 189
    and "holistic methods," 31
    and nutrition, 35
Chlorophyll, 66
Cholesterol, 172, 189
    blood levels, 173-174, 176
    dietary recommendations,
        175-176
    and heart disease, 171, 173
    sources, 172-173
Choline, 29, 66
Chorionic gonadotropin, human
    (HCG), 120, 130*t*
Chromium, GTF, 72-73
Chyme, 7
Cider vinegar, 66
Cigarette smoking, cancer risk, 182
Clinical ecology, 32-33, 189
Cocoa, caffeine content, 154*t*
Coconut oil, 10
"Coffee nerves," 152
Coffee, and pancreatic cancer, 153
"Cold pressed" oils, 66-67
Colitis, 189
Colon, functions, 7
Committee for Freedom of Choice
    in Medicine, 41

Computer analysis of diet, 35-36, 37
Computers, for diet planning, 35-36
Confederation of Health Organizations, 41
Congeners, in alcoholic beverages, 155
Consulting Nutritionists, 38
Consumer Health Education Council, 44
Consumer Reports, 42*t*, 49, 67
Controlled experiment, 189
Coronary heart disease (CHD), 171-175
Cosmetics
  "hypoallergenic," 85
  "natural," 85
Council for Agricultural Science and Technology, 41
Council for Postsecondary Accreditation, 40
Council for Responsible Nutrition, 36, 41
Council of Better Business Bureaus, National Advertising Division, 46
Crook, Dr. William, 83
Cyclamate, 189

Delaney Clause, 102
Dental hygiene, 147
Desiccated liver, 67
Desirable weight, 111-112, 112*t*, 189-190
"Detoxification" of body, 29
Diabetes, 190
  fructose in, 145
  and sugar consumption, 144
Diagnostic tests, dubious
  bogus computer analysis, 35
  hair analysis, 34-35
  "Nutrient Deficiency Test," 39
  provocation and neutralization, 33
  vitamin questionnaires, 37-37
Diamond, Harvey and Marilyn, 126

Diathermy, 190
Diet(s)
  advice on, 37-38
  for athletes, 168
  balancing, 16-18, 18*t*-19*t*
  and cancer, 63, 180-184
  computer analysis, 35-36, 37
  crash, to lower weight for athletic events, 167
  Feingold, 105-106
  and heart disease, 171-180
  liquid protein, 119
  low-fat, 114-115
  macrobiotic, 138-139
  "magic diet" myth, 30
  popular, 126, 128*t*-131*t*
  Pritikin, 179-180
  protein-sparing modified fast, 119
  sensible, 127
  U.S., changes in, 24-25, 94, 174-175
  vegetarian; *see* Vegetarian diets
  very-low-calorie, 119
  vitamin supplementation not needed, 123
Diet aids
  nonprescription, 121-123
  prescription, 120
Diet and Health, 20
Diet books, typical characteristics, 126
Diet Center Diet, 128*t*
Diet clinics, 115
Diet industry, scope of, 110
Diet, Nutrition, and Cancer, 180
Diet planning, computers for, 35-36
Diet Workshop Diet, 116, 129*t*
Dietary guidelines
  for adults, 20
  for children, 20-22
Dietary problem, in U.S., 25
"Dieters' worst enemies," 22, 114
Dietitians, 37-39, 190
Digestion, 5, 7
Diuretics, 56
Diverticulosis, 182

Dolomite, 59, 67
Donsbach University, 39
Donsbach, Kurt, 39
Dr. Stillman's Quick Weight-Loss
     Diet, 129t
Drinking Man's Diet, 129t
Drunkenness, development of, 157
Dublin, Louis, 111

East West Foundation, 138
Eating patterns, in U.S., 24-25,
     94, 174-175
EDTA, disodium, 32
Efamol, Ltd., 68
Eggs
     fertilized, 68-69
     significance of shell color, 69
Emulsifier, 190
Energy, from protein sources,
     23-24
Energy
     food; *see* Calories
     "quick," 144, 169
     storage forms of, 8-9
Enforcement actions
     "anti-cancer supplements," 184
     "anti-yeast" products, 83
     evening primrose oil, 68
     fish oils, 69
     germanium, 69
     green-lipped mussel, 72
     octacosanol, 77
     "oral chelation" products, 77
     raw milk, 79
     "starch blockers," 122
     "stress vitamins," 49-50
     "vitamin B$_{15}$," 81
Enrichment, 190
Environmental contaminants in
     foods, 99
Enzymes, 190
     digestive, 5, 7, 78
     oral, 67-68, 81
     pancreatic, 7
Eosinophilia-myalgia syndrome, 63
Epidemiology, 190
Erewhon Natural Foods Company,

138
"Ergogenic aids," 68, 83
Esophagus, 5
Ethylenediamine tetra-acetic acid
     (EDTA), 32
Evening primrose oil, 68
Exchange lists, 190
Exercise
     eating prior to, 169
     "passive," 124, 125
     and weight control, 114

F-Plan Diet, 129t
"Fast foods"
     calorie content, 92
     definition of, 88, 191
     nutritional value of, 88-89, 88t,
          92-93
     popularity of, 88
     in school cafeterias, 92-94
     selection of nutritious meal,
          89-90, 91-92
Fasting, 84, 129t, 118
     modified ("protein-sparing"),
          119
Fat(s), 2, 9-10, 191
     as source of calories, 23
     body, essential functions, 113
     diets high in, and cancer, 184
     hidden, 23
     in meats, 23t
     monounsaturated, 9, 175, 194
     polyunsaturated, 9, 175, 195
     recommendations for infants, 21
     saturated, 9, 175, 196
     unsaturated, 9, 175, 197
Fat-Destroyer Foods Diet, 129t
Fatigue, unrelated to nutrition, 24
Fatty acids, 9-10, 191
FDA; *see* Food and Drug
     Administration
Federal Trade Commission (FTC),
     45
     food advertising rule, 11
     and "stress vitamins," 49-50
Feingold diet, 105-106
Fenfluramine, 120

Fertilized eggs, 68-69
Fetal alcohol syndrome, 159-160
Fiber pills, 183
Fiber, dietary, 8, 176, 191
   recommendations for infants, 21
   and zinc deficiency, 56
Fish oils, 69
Fit for Life Diet, 126, 129*t*
Fluid needs, for athletes, 168
Fluoridation, 147, 191
Fluoride
   and mottling of teeth, 13
   and osteoporosis, 54
   supplements, 13, 54
   and tooth decay, 13
Folic acid, 48
Food(s)
   additives; *see* Additives
   choices, in U.S., 24-25, 94,
      174-175
   enrichment, 190
   "fast"; *see* "Fast foods"
   fortification, 191
   hazards, 99
   "health"; *see* "Health foods"
   highest in sodium, 177-178
   "junk"; *see* "Junk foods"
   labels, 4-5
   "light," 117
   "natural"; *see* "natural" foods
   natural toxicants in, 99
   number in typical supermarket,
      17
   "organically grown," 11, 28,
      77-78, 195
   safety, 28, 101-102
   snack, 84
Food and Drug Administration
      (FDA), 42
   and food additives, 97-98
   and food labels, 4-5
   and homeopathic remedies, 75
   jurisdiction, 45
   as target of quacks, 29
   see also Enforcement actions
Food and Nutrition Board, 3, 95
   196

Food combining, 191
Food faddist, 190-191
Food irradiation, 107, 191
Food Protection Committee, 95
Food supplements, 61, 191
Fortification, 191
Foundation for the Advancement
      of Innovative Medicine, 41
Framingham Heart Study, 173
Fredrick, Len, 92-93
Fructose, 118, 142, 145, 191
Fructose Diet, 129*t*

Galactose, 8, 191
Gamma-linoleic acid (GLA), 68
Garlic, 69
"Gas," foods causing, 62
Gastric stapling, 124
Gastrointestinal tract, 5-7
Gerber Products Company, 20, 22
Germanium, 69-70
Gerovital H3 (GH3), 61, 70
Ginkgo biloba, 70
Ginseng, 70
Glandular extracts, 71
Glucomannan, 121
Glucose, 8, 191
Glutamic acid, 71
Glycogen, 9, 191
Goat milk, 71-72
Goiter, 55, 191
Gout, 191
Granola, 72
Grapefruit Diet, 129*t*
GRAS list, 98
Great Earth Vitamin Stores, 36-37
Green-lipped mussel, 72
"Growth hormone releasers,"
      122-123, 170
GTF chromium, 72-73
Guar gum, 122
Gums, 191
Gymnema sylvestre, 73

Hair analysis, 34-35
Hall, Richard, 100
HCG Diet, 120, 130*t*

HDL, 173-174, 176, 192
   and alcohol intake, 159
"Health clubs," 124
"Health food(s)," 84, 85-86
   as slogan, 11
   definition, 61, 192
   nutrients in, 61, 86
   promotion and prices of, 61
"Health food" industry, 26
"Health food" stores
   advice at, 44-45
   and weight-loss products,
      121-122
Heart disease
   and alcoholic intake, 159
   and caffeine, 153
   and diet, 171-180
   prevention, 179
   risk factors, 173, 179
   and sugar consumption,
      145-146, 179
   and water hardness, 160
Herbal teas, 74t, 154
Herbalife, 130t
Herbert, Dr. Victor, 27
Herbs
   adverse effects of, 74t
   "health food" stores sales, 73
High-density lipoproteins; *see* HDL
"Holistic" health care, 31-32, 192
Homeopathic remedies, 74-75
Homeopathy, 33-34, 74, 192
Honey, 74, 148
Hormone, definition of, 192
Human chorionic gonadotropin
      (HCG), 120
Huxley Institute for Biosocial
      Research, 41
Hydrogenation, 10, 192
Hyperactivity, 192
   additives and, 105-106
   sugar and, 146-147
Hyperalimentation, 192
Hypercholesterolemia, 192
Hyperkalemia, 56
Hyperkinesis; *see* hyperactivity

Hypertension, 192
   sodium and, 14
Hypnosis, to reduce appetite, 123
Hypoglycemia, 145, 192

I Love New York Diet, 130t
"Immune boosters," 83
Information sources
   nonrecommended, 40-41, 42, 43t
   recommended, 41-42, 42t-43t
Inositol, 29, 75
Institute of Food Technologists, 41
Insulin, 192
Intermittent claudication, 32
International Academy of Nutrition
      and Preventive Medicine, 41
International Association of Cancer
      Victors and Friends, 41
International Association of
      Dentists and Physicians, 41
International Life Sciences
      Institute—Nutrition
      Foundation, 42
International University for
      Nutrition Education, 39
Intestinal bypass, 124
Intestines, 7
Iodide, amounts in diet, 55
Iridology, 39, 193
Iron
   absorption, 12
   deficiency, 12, 169
   functions, 12
   recommendations for infants, 21
   sources, 12, 22, 53, 136t
   supplements, 53, 54
Irradiation, food, 107

Jarvis, Dr. William, T., 27, 60
Jaw wiring, 124
"Junk food(s)," 87, 143-144, 193

Kefir, 61
Kelp, 75-76
Kelp, Lecithin, Vitamin B$_6$, and
      Cider Vinegar Diet, 130t

Kilocalorie, 188
Kinesiology, applied, 31
Kushi, Michio, 138

L-lysine, 77
L-tryptophan, 63
Lact-Aid, 61-62
Lactation, 59, 193
Lactose intolerance, 61-62, 193
Lactose, 8, 193
Laetrile, 29, 61, 76, 193
Last Chance Diet, 119, 130*t*
LDL, 173-174, 176, 193
Lecithin, 61, 76, 193
Lederle Laboratories, 49
Legumes, 193
Life Extension Foundation, 41
Life Extension, 82
"Light" foods, 117
Lignin, 193
Linoleic acid, 9, 193
Lipids, 193; *see also* Fat(s)
Lipoproteins, 193; *see also* HDL;
    LDL
Liposuction, 125
Liquid protein diets, 130*t*
Liver, desiccated, 67
Low blood sugar, 145, 192
Low-density proteins; *see* LDL

Macrobiotic diet, 138-139, 193
Macronutrients, 3*t*
Maltose, 194
March of Dimes Foundation, 160
Massage, 124
Mayo Diet, 130*t*
Mazindol, 120
Meats, fat content, 23*t*
Medicine, "holistic," 31-32, 192
Megadose, 194
Megaloblastic anemia, 194
Megavitamin therapy," 50
Metabolism, 194
Microbiological hazards in foods,
    99
Microminerals, 12

Micronutrients, 3*t*
Miles Laboratories, 49-50
Milk
    "certified," 79
    goat, 71-72
    raw (unpasteurized), 79
Minerals, 11-14, 194
    chelated, 65-66
    effect of cooking, 53
    essential, 3*t*, 12
    functions, 11
    significant for consumers, 12
    sources, 54
    supplements, 53-59
    toxic effects, 54
    trace, 12
Misinformation, spread of, 26-27
Molasses, 149
    blackstrap, 64
Mono-food diets, 130*t*
Monosodium glutamate (MSG),
    107-108
Morbid obesity, 123-124
MSG, 107-108
Myocardial infarction, 172

National Academy of Sciences
    and Delaney Clause, 102
    diet-cancer guidelines, 63,
    180-181
National Council Against Health
    Fraud, 42, 46
National Health Federation, 41
National Nutritional Foods
    Association, 41
National Research Council, 20,
    95, 185, 196
"Natural foods," 11, 28, 99-102,
    194
Naturopathy, 34, 194
Niacin, 48, 176
Nitrates/nitrites 104-105
Nitrosamines, 104-105, 158
Nucleic acids, 194
"Nutrient Deficiency Test," 39
Nutri/System, 130*t*

Nutrients
  "anti-aging," 82-83
  basic categories, 3t
  and calories, 3
  essential, 2-4, 3t, 190
  "optimal" amounts, 4
  providing food energy, 3
Nutrition
  advice, where to seek, 2, 37-38
  for athletes, 22, 168-169
  basics, 1-15
  definition, 194
  education of children, 93-94
  good, basic rules of, 1
  information, evaluation of, 26-45
  information sources, 40-43, 43t
  misinformation, spread of, 26-27
  past vs. present, 16
  quackery; see Quackery
  scams, reporting of, 45-46
  tips for teenagers, 161-170
Nutrition for Optimal Health
  Association, 41
"Nutrition insurance," 28-29, 49, 50
Nutritionists
  checking credentials, 40
  legitimate, 37-39, 194
  unqualified, 28, 40

Oat bran, 64-65
Obesity
  definition, 110-111, 195
  hazards, 111
  morbid, 123-124
  risk for cancer, 182
  surgery for, 123-124
Octacosanol, 77
Oils, 9-10
  "cold pressed," 66-67
Omnivorous, 195
"Oral chelation" products, 77
"Organically grown" foods, 11, 28,
  77-78, 195
Organizations, for nutrition advice
  reliable, 41-42
  questionable, 40-41
Orthomolecular Medical Society, 41

Orthomolecular therapy, 50
Osteomalacia, 13, 195
Osteoporosis, 13, 195
  calcium and, 55
  fluoride and, 54
Overnutrition, as problem in U.S.,
  87
Overweight, and overfat,
  compared, 113-114, 195

PABA, 29, 61, 78
Palm oil, 10
Pancreas, 7
Pangamate, 29, 81
Pangamic acid, 81
Papain, 78
Para-aminobenzoic acid (PABA),
  29, 61, 78
"Passion flower" fruit, 78-79
Passive exercise, 124, 125
Pauling, Linus, 51
Pearson, Durk, 82-83
Pectin, 122, 195
Pellagra, 25, 195
People's Medical Society, 41
Pesticides, 99, 108-109, 195
Phenylketonuria, 103-104
Phenylpropanolamine (PPA), 121
Phospholipids, 195
Physiology, 195
Plaque (arterial), 195
Postal Service, jurisdiction of, 45
Postmenopausal, 195
Potassium
  blood pressure, 178
  deficiency, 14
  excess, 14
  foods rich in, 57t
  role of, 14
  supplements, 14, 56
Pregnancy, and alcohol
  consumption, 159-160
Precursor, 189
Preservatives, 195
Price-Pottenger Nutrition
  Foundation, 41
Pritikin Diet, 179-180

Procaine, 70
Project Cure, 41
Proof, of alcoholic beverages,
    155-156
Protein supplements, 79
Protein(s), 7-8, 196
    for athletes, 22, 168-169
    complete, 136
    composition, 2-3, 7
    as energy sources, 23-24
    functions, 8
    synthetic vegetable, 137-138
    for vegetarians, 135, 136*t*,
        137-138
Protein-sparing diets, 119
Proteins, complete, 135, 136*t*
Provocation and neutralization test,
    33
Pseudonutritionists, 196

Quacks, 27, 196
Quackery
    cost of, 60
    definition, 27, 196
    doctors and, 31
    information sources, 41-42
    promotion, 26-27
    vulnerability to, 30-31
    ways to recognize, 27-30
"Quick energy," 144, 169

Raw milk, 79
Raw sugar, 148
RDAs; *see* Recommended Dietary
    Allowances
RDIs; *see* Reference Daily Intakes
Rebound scurvy, 48
Recommended Daily Allowances,
    U.S., 4-5
Recommended Dietary Allowances
    (RDAs), 3-4, 5, 185*t*-186*t*,
    196
Reference Daily Intakes (RDIs), 5
Reflexology, 31, 196
Riboflavin, sources, 136*t*
Rice Diet, 130*t*
Rickets, 13, 24, 138, 196

Risk factors, 196
    for cancer, 182-183
    for coronary heart disease, 173,
        179
RNA/DNA supplements, 79
Rose hips, vitamin C from, 52
Rotation Diet, 131*t*
Royal jelly, 80
Rutin, 80

Saccharin, 102-103, 104
Salt pills, for athletes, 170
Salt substitutes, 56
Sampson, Wallace I., 32
Saunas, 124
Scarsdale Diet, 131*t*
Scientific method, 2
Scurvy, 24, 196
    rebound, 48
Sea salt, 80
"Seawater concentrates," 80
Selenium, 58
Shaklee Corporation, 26
Shampoos, "organic," 85
Shaw, Sandy, 82-83
Silicon, 58
Ski Team Diet, 131*t*
Snacks, for children, 93
Sodium, 197
    foods highest in, 177-178
    functions, 14
    and heart disease, 177-178
    and high blood pressure, 14
    recommendations for infants, 21
    restriction, 177-178
    "sensitivity," 14
    in softened water, 160-161
Southampton Diet, 131*t*
Spirulina, 80, 122
"Spot-reducing," 125
Sprouts, 81
"Starch blockers," 122
Starches, 196-197
Steroid drugs, 170
Sterol, 197
Stomach cancer, and BHA and
    BHT, 106-107

Stomach, "shrinking," 118
"Stress vitamins," 28, 49-50
Submarine sandwiches, 90
Sucrose, 197
Sugar
    accusations against, 142-144,
        146-147
    "addiction," 146
    and behavior, 146-147
    brown, 148-149
    consumption/disappearance,
        142-142
    and diabetes, 144-145
    as "fun food," 144
    and heart disease, 145-146, 179
    "raw," 148
    recommendations for infants, 21
    safety, 143
    simple, 8
    substitutes, 102-104
    and tooth decay, 147
    truth about, 30, 142-149
    turbinado, 148
Sulfites, 108
Superoxide dismutase (SOD), 81
Supplements
    "anti-cancer," 183-184
    for athletes, 169, 170
*Surgeon General's Report on
    Nutrition and Health,* 20
Sweeteners, artificial, 102-104

Tea
    alfalfa, 62
    caffeine in, 153-154, 154*t*
    herbal, 73, 73*t*
Testimonials, quacks and, 29
Textured vegetable protein (TVP),
    137-138
The 35-Plus Diet for Women, 131*t*
Thyroid gland, 197
Thyroid hormones, in weight
    reduction, 120
Tired blood," 12
Tooth decay
    fluoride and, 13

soft drinks and, 147-148
sugar and, 147
TOPS, 115, 116
Toxicants, natural, in foods, 99
Triglyceride(s), 9-10, 197
Turbinado sugar, 148, 197

U.S. RDAs (U.S. Recommended
    Daily Allowances), 4-5
University Diet, 131*t*
Urethane, 158-159

Vegan diet, disadvantages, 138
Vegetarian diet(s), 132-140
    advantages, 140
    balancing of, 133, 134
    food volume needed, 137
    protein sources, 134-135, 136*t*
    sources of important nutrients,
        136*t*
    reasons for choosing, 133
    main types, 132
    tips for constructing, 140
    and vitamin B_{12} supplements,
        137
Vending machines, in schools,
    148
Very-low-calorie diets, 119
Vitamin A
    excess, symptoms of, 47-48
    sources, 50-51
    synthetic, anticancer activity, 51
Vitamin B_6, excess, dangers of, 48
Vitamin B_{12}
    deficiency, symptoms of, 137
    supplements for vegetarians,
        137
"Vitamin B_{15}," 29
"Vitamin B_{17}," 29, 76
Vitamin C
    and cancer, 52
    and common cold, 51
    excess, dangers of, 48
    "natural," 52
    and nitrites, 105
    sources of, 52, 79, 136*t*

Vitamin D
  excess, dangers of, 48
  sources, 136
Vitamin E
  and breast lumps, 52
  and "cold pressed" oils, 67
  excess, symptoms of, 48
  and sexual vigor, 53
  sources, 66, 67
"Vitamin F," 82
Vitamin Gap" Test, 36, 46
"Vitamin P," 64
Vitamins, 10-11
  composition, 3
  fat-soluble, 10-11
  functions, 10
  misconceptions, 24, 47
  "natural" vs. synthetic, 28, 29
  phony, 29
  questionnaires, 36-37
  "stress," 28, 49-50
  supplements, 47-53, 123
  toxicity, 47-48
  water-soluble, 10, 11

Water
  bottled, 160-161
  fluoridated, 147, 191
  in foods, 15
  functions, 14-15
  health effects of softness and
    hardness, 160-161
  requirements, daily, 24
Weight
  for athletic competition,
    167

  desirable, 111-112, 112t,
  calories and, 113-114
    189-190
  excess, hazards of, 111
    189-190
  "ideal," 189
Weight control, 110-131; *see also*
    Diet(s); Fasting
  and artificial sweeteners, 104
  behavioral modification tips,
    115-116
  and exercise, 114
  and "light" foods, 117
  most sensible plan, 114-115
  program evaluation, 116
  for teenagers, 161-163
  tips for college students, 117
  vitamin supplementation
    while dieting, 123
Weight loss
  as national obsession, 110
  products; *see* Diet aids
  surgical procedures, 123-124
Weight Watchers, 115, 116
"Wellness" centers, 31-32
Wheat germ, 82
World Research Foundation,
    41

Yeast Connection, The, 83
Yeast infections, 83
Yeast, brewer's, 65
"Yo-yo dieting," 167
Yogurt, 61, 82

Zinc, 56